Understanding

Health Outcomes and Pharmacoeconomics

George E. MacKinnon III, PhD, RPh, FASHP

Principal, HealthKey Solutions, Inc.
Founding Dean and Professor
College of Pharmacy
Roosevelt University
Schaumburg Campus
Schaumburg, IL

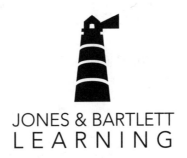

JONES & BARTLETT
LEARNING

World Headquarters
Jones & Bartlett Learning
5 Wall Street
Burlington, MA 01803
978-443-5000
info@jblearning.com
www.jblearning.com

Jones & Bartlett Learning books and products are available through most bookstores and online booksellers. To contact Jones & Bartlett Learning directly, call 800-832-0034, fax 978-443-8000, or visit our website, www.jblearning.com.

Production Credits

Publisher: David D. Cella
Acquisitions Editor: Katey Birtcher
Managing Editor: Maro Gartside
Editorial Assistant: Teresa Reilly
Senior Production Editor: Renée Sekerak
Production Assistant: Sean Coombs
Marketing Manager: Grace Richards
Manufacturing and Inventory Control
   Supervisor: Amy Bacus

Composition: Cenveo Publisher Services
Cover Images: Business chart © Sergey
   Khakimullin/Dreamstime.com; Assortment of
   pills © Andrzej Tokarski/Dreamstime.com
Printing and Binding: Malloy, Inc.
Cover Printing: Malloy, Inc.

Library of Congress Cataloging-in-Publication Data
  Understanding health outcomes and pharmacoeconomics / edited by George E. MacKinnon III.
    p. ; cm.
  Includes bibliographical references and index.
  ISBN 978-0-7637-7099-0 (pbk. : alk. paper) 1. Pharmaceutical industry—Economic aspects.
2. Drugs—Cost effectiveness. 3. Drug development—Economic aspects. 4. Outcome Assessment (Health Care) I. MacKinnon, George E.
  [DNLM: 1. Economics, Pharmaceutical. 2. Costs and Cost Analysis—methods. 3. Outcome Assessment (Health Care)—economics. QV 736]
  RS100.U53 2012
  338.4'76151—dc23
                2011022068

6048
Printed in the United States of America
15 14 13 12 11   10 9 8 7 6 5 4 3 2 1

Dedication

To my wife and children who have endured the countless hours taken from them by me overseeing the research and production of this work—not to mention "the dinners" which have included a healthy serving of pharmaceuticals, a side of health care, and a dash of politics on any given evening.

To my parents who inspired the drive in me to always do my best professionally and personally.

Acknowledgments

I would like to recognize the students who over the years have inspired and challenged me in the classroom, in practice, and in life. Likewise there have been colleagues within higher education, the health sciences and clinical practice communities, the health insurance industry, as well as the pharmaceutical industry that have provided sage knowledge and guidance to me.

I would like to thank the entire team at Jones & Bartlett Learning, in particular, the publisher, David D. Cella, for listening to my ideas some years back on the creation of this resource for healthcare students and practitioners alike. I would be remiss if I did not acknowledge Maro Gartside and Katey Birtcher for their patience with deadlines and the editorial and production assistance of Teresa Reilly, Renée Sekerak, and Sapna Rastogi. Lastly this book would not have been possible without the contributions and efforts of the chapter authors, who in their own right have advanced my understanding of the concepts and materials, as I hope occurs for others as they use the resources provided.

Contents

CHAPTER 3 ▪ Measuring Health Status and Health-Related Quality-of-Life Assessment   25

Nalin Payakachat, BPharm, MSc, PhD
Matthew M. Murawski, BPharm, PhD

CHAPTER 4 ▪ Health Surveys (Disease-Specific and Generic Questionnaires) and Utility Assessment   39

Patricia van Hanswijck de Jonge, PhD
Donald E. Stull, PhD

CHAPTER 5 ■ Overview of Statistical Analysis in Biomedical Research   57

Chenghui Li, PhD

SECTION II ■ Evaluating Levels of Evidence   83

CHAPTER 6 ■ Randomized Controlled Trials   85

Nathaniel M. Rickles, PharmD, PhD, BCPP
Matthew Wolfe, BA

CHAPTER 9 ■ Uses of Real-World Data in Evidence Development   **139**

Carl V. Asche, PhD

SECTION III ■ Pharmacoeconomics

CHAPTER 13 ■ Cost-Effectiveness Analysis, Cost-Utility Analysis, and Cost-Benefit Analysis   179

Junhua Yu, PhD
Jaewhan Kim, PhD

CHAPTER 14 ■ Comparative Effectiveness   195

Patrick D. Meek, PharmD, MSPH
Amy C. Renaud-Mutart, PharmD, MSPharm
Leon E. Cosler, RPh, PhD

Foreword

Following my pharmacy clinical residency, I chose a path very different from many of my pharmacy peers—I pursued a fellowship in Pharmacoeconomics. I was driven by my clinical research demonstrating the benefits of a newly marketed product, Epogen, on patients' quality of life. Witnessing positive changes in physical and emotional endpoints in conjunction with the improvements seen in the traditional clinical markers for these patients receiving dialysis, I knew immediately the cost of this drug was worth every penny. From this experience, I was determined to pursue a research career demonstrating the value of effectiveness, safety, health, and economic endpoints together in order to drive more informed decisions regarding the allocation of healthcare dollars.

The educational tools at the time were limited to a primer, which provided the definitions and analytical basis for conducting pharmacoeconomic research. What was missing from the literature was the application of these theories and equations for pharmacists. To bridge theory to practice, I published an article, "Guidelines for Performing a Pharmacoeconomic Analysis," in an attempt to encourage pharmacists and other medical providers to conduct their own research in this area. This was a good start, but I was unaware that this research field was about to take off—and it did. Almost every pharmaceutical company and payer organization added a research arm responsible for demonstrating value, and pharmacy schools began to add the topic of pharmacoeconomics to the curriculum.

Over the last 20 years, the study and importance of pharmacoeconomics, health outcomes, health economics, and epidemiology have grown along with the increased demand for evidence beyond the traditional safety and efficacy endpoints. The true tipping point in the United States came with the signing of the American Recovery and Reinvestment Act of 2009 (ARRA) where the term comparative effectiveness research (CER) became known by all healthcare researchers and providers. This milestone elevated the importance for all healthcare providers and payers to better understand the techniques and tools for comparing not only pharmaceutical products but all interventions in relation to conventional treatment.

This textbook is intended to provide pharmacists and other healthcare providers with a comprehensive overview and applicable tools in order to conduct research demonstrating value to both the patient and the healthcare system. As pharmacists, we have the opportunity to lead this research as we practice across the various care settings. We are consulted and relied on to recommend and distribute biopharmaceuticals—where spending on medicines can lead to decreased hospitalization costs and extended life expectancy—but only if we have the evidence that can be applied at point of care. Therefore, we should call upon ourselves as healthcare providers to learn how to best assess new interventions and treatments. Dr. MacKinnon and the contributing authors have prepared a premier textbook that will be your foundation for conducting new and applicable health outcomes and pharmacoeconomic research.

Lynn Jolicoeur Okamoto, PharmD
Senior Vice President, Health Economics
United BioSource Corporation

Lynn J. Okamoto, PharmD is Senior Vice President of Health Economics and a Senior Research Scientist at United BioSource Corporation (UBC) in Bethesda, Maryland. Dr. Okamoto leads the health economic and policy efforts in the United States and interfaces with UBC's European operations on global issues. She has extensive experience in global management, as well as advanced leadership skills and command of strategic planning and implementation.

Dr. Okamoto has well over a decade of experience conducting health outcomes and pharmacoeconomic research and has held senior-level positions at NDCHealth and Glaxo Wellcome. She assisted in developing domestic and international pharmacoeconomic research strategy for various pharmaceutical products.

During her tenure at Glaxo Wellcome, Dr. Okamoto took an active role in pharmacoeconomic research at many levels, including decision modeling, strategic health outcomes research in support of new products, and regulatory strategy. Bringing this expertise to NDCHealth, she created and directed the company's Outcomes Research department. In her most recent position at NDCHealth, Dr. Okamoto served as Vice President and General Manager of the Intelligent Health Repository.

Dr. Okamoto received her Doctor of Pharmacy from the University of Michigan, and her work in pharmacoeconomics has led to publication in healthcare journals, including *Clinical Therapeutics*, the *Journal of Asthma*, *Pharmacotherapy*, the *American Journal of Managed Care*, and the *Annals of Allergy, Asthma & Immunology*. Her research covers a wide variety of therapeutic areas and perspectives, from cost-of-illness analyses in respiratory care and influenza management, to quality-of-life studies in asthma. Dr. Okamoto's research has been exhibited internationally at conferences such as the International Society of Pharmacoeconomic and Outcomes Research Annual & European Conferences, and the European Respiratory Society Annual Congress.

Contributors

Carl V. Asche, MBA, PhD
Director
Professor of Medicine
Center for Health Outcomes Research
University of Illinois College of Medicine Peoria
Peoria, IL

Leon E. Cosler, RPh, PhD
Associate Professor
Department of Pharmacy Practice and Research Institute for Health Outcomes
Albany College of Pharmacy and Health Sciences
Albany, NY

Patricia M. Finnegan, MS
Pharmaceutical Industry Consultant
Glenview, IL

Jaewhan Kim, PhD
Assistant Professor
Division of Public Health
Department of Family and Preventive Medicine
University of Utah
Salt Lake City, UT

Donald G. Klepser, PhD, MBA
Assistant Professor
Department of Pharmacy Practice
College of Pharmacy
University of Nebraska Medical Center
Omaha, NE

Chenghui Li, PhD
Division of Pharmaceutical Evaluation and Policy
College of Pharmacy
University of Arkansas for Medical Sciences
Little Rock, AR

Steven E. Marx, RPh, PharmD
Director
Global Health Economics and Outcomes Research
Abbott Laboratories
Abbott Park, IL

Patrick D. Meek, PharmD, MSPH
Assistant Professor of Pharmacy
Department of Pharmacy Practice and Research Institute for Health Outcomes
Albany College of Pharmacy and Health Sciences
Albany, NY

Matthew M. Murawski, BPharm, PhD
Department of Pharmacy Practice
Purdue University School of Pharmacy and Pharmaceutical Sciences
West Lafayette, IN

Nalin Payakachat, BPharm, MSc, PhD
Division of Pharmaceutical Evaluation and Policy
College of Pharmacy
University of Arkansas for Medical Sciences
Little Rock, AR

Amy C. Renaud-Mutart, PharmD
Assistant Professor
Department of Pharmacy Practice and Research Institute for Health Outcomes
Albany College of Pharmacy and Health Sciences
Albany, NY

Nathaniel M. Rickles, PharmD, PhD, BCPP
Associate Professor of Pharmacy Practice and Administration
Bouve College of Health Sciences
School of Pharmacy
Northeastern University
Boston, MA

Gerald E. Schumacher, PharmD, MSc, PhD
Professor of Pharmacy Emeritus
Bouve College of Health Sciences
School of Pharmacy
Northeastern University
Boston, MA

Donald E. Stull, PhD
Director
Retrospective Data Analysis
RTI Health Solutions
Manchester, UK

Patricia van Hanswijck de Jonge, PhD
United BioSource Corporation
London, UK

Matthew Wolfe, BA (PharmD Candidate)
School of Pharmacy
Temple University
Philadelphia, PA

Junhua Yu, PhD
Assistant Professor
Department of Social Behavior and Administrative Sciences
Touro University College of Pharmacy
Vallejo, CA

Reviewers

Grace M. Kuo, PharmD, MPH
Associate Professor of Clinical Pharmacy
Associate Adjunct Professor of Family and Preventive Medicine
University of California, San Diego
La Jolla, CA

David J. Mihm, RPh, PhD
Assistant Professor
Division of Clinical and Administrative Science
College of Pharmacy
Xavier University of Louisiana
New Orleans, LA

Stephanie C. Peshek, PharmD, MBA, FASHP
Assistant Professor of Pharmacy Practice
School of Pharmacy
The Lake Erie College of Osteopathic Medicine
Bradenton, FL

Hong Xiao, PhD
Professor and Director
Division of Economic, Social, and Administrative Pharmacy
College of Pharmacy and Pharmaceutical Sciences
Florida Agricultural and Mechanical University
Tallahassee, FL

About the Author

A native of northern Wisconsin, Dr. George E. MacKinnon III received both his BS (Pharmacy) and MS (Hospital Pharmacy) from the University of Wisconsin–Madison. He completed two years of postgraduate clinical pharmacy residency training at the University of Wisconsin Hospital and Clinics. He obtained his PhD in Educational Leadership and Policy Studies from Loyola University Chicago. Over the past 20 years, he has held joint academic appointments in medicine and pharmacy at various educational institutions engaging in clinical practice, research, teaching, and academic administration. His previous appointments include Vice President of Academic Affairs with the American Association of Colleges of Pharmacy in Alexandria, Virginia, and Director of Global Health Economics and Outcomes Research of Abbott Laboratories.

Dr. MacKinnon has been involved in a leadership capacity in the establishment and subsequent accreditation of three new colleges of pharmacy in the United States (Chicago and Phoenix). Dr. MacKinnon has engaged in significant curricular innovation (accelerated graduation and nontraditional pathways; integrated curriculum of biological, clinical, and pharmaceutical sciences; and use of student annual academic assessments) with respect to the professional doctor of pharmacy degree (PharmD). He taught one of the first required courses in pharmacoeconomics, health economics, and outcomes assessment at an academic pharmacy program in the early 1990s.

Dr. MacKinnon has assisted in the development of numerous pharmacist–medical practice initiatives as well as several postgraduate residency training programs in various practice settings over the years. He led the development of academic-practice partnerships that have been modeled across the United States. Dr. MacKinnon's personal research interests and developed products relate to documenting the value of pharmacists' and students' interventions with patients and other healthcare providers, and demonstrating the overall clinical and economic impact of such encounters to stakeholders. He has secured extramural funding in excess of $1.2 million to support various educational programs and research projects.

Dr. MacKinnon served as the Founding Editor of *InetCE* [SM], one of the first Internet-based continuing education publications, from 1996–2006. Dr. MacKinnon has delivered over 220 presentations, written over 60 publications, and authored several book chapters in pharmacy and the health sciences arena. He received the Clinical Faculty Award for Teaching from the 1992 graduating PharmD class of the St. Louis College of Pharmacy. In 2000, he was recognized by peers as a Fellow of the American Society of Health–System Pharmacists (FASHP), and in 2003, he was the recipient of the Service to Pharmacy Award from the Arizona Pharmacists Association.

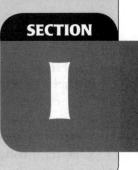

Introduction to Measuring Health Status

We begin with an overview of the issues surrounding escalating health care costs, competitive technologies and new products, increased availability of medical and prescription data, health-related quality-of-life (HRQL) issues, and finite resources to cover the escalating health care costs in Chapter 1. Although determining what the benefits and costs are may seem obvious, their identification can be challenging. Clinical trials are very useful, but they have some inherent weaknesses such as limited number and range of subjects, use of surrogate end points, lack of active comparators (often compared to a placebo), relative limited time frame for the study, and the absence of risk-benefit analysis. The ultimate goal is for decision makers and health care providers to make evidence-based clinical decisions for patients with quality improvement as a constant.

The drug approval process in the United States has been evolutionary yet political from focusing initially on safety through the Federal Food, Drug and Cosmetic (FFDC) Act of 1938 to encompassing efficacy in drug approval reviews following passage of the Kefauver-Harris Drug Amendments in 1962. Drugs, biological products, and medical devices sold in the United States are regulated by the Food and Drug Administration (FDA), a government agency within the Department of Health and Human Services (DHHS). Public pressure to bring new medications to patients faster led to the passage of the Hatch-Waxman Amendments to the FFDC Act in 1984, allowing manufacturers of generic drugs to rely on findings of safety and efficacy of the previously approved drug, and the Prescription Drug User Fee Act (PDUFA) of 1992, authorizing the collection of fees from pharmaceutical manufacturers for regulatory submissions to the FDA. However, public pressure to bring new medications to patients faster and rising costs of drug development exist not only in the United States but in other countries as well. Chapter 2 concludes with a discussion of the challenges associated with the advent of biologics (large molecules) and the subsequent development of biosimilars. These biotechnology developments led to the Patient Protection and Affordable Care (PPAC) Act, also called the Biologics Price Competition and Innovation (BPCI) Act, in 2010.

As described in Chapter 3, HRQL is an important element that has seen increased attention in the health care decision-making processes, not only to inform physicians regarding treatment outcomes (both favorable and unfavorable) but also to assist policy makers to better allocate limited health care resources. Both generic and disease-specific HRQL measurement instruments are used to assess the different domains of health including physical, psychological, role and social, disease-specific functioning, and general health perceptions. In clinical practice, health care providers may use HRQL assessments or the results from their use in clinical trials to maximize patient outcomes from treatments.

Chapter 4 continues the discussion of measuring health and HRQL via generic or disease-specific, patient-reported or clinician-assessed instruments. Valuing health involves establishing the relative value or importance people (eg, patients or the general public) place on different dimensions of health, different levels of each dimension of health, and different combinations of levels of dimensions (ie, health states). This chapter provides various examples of techniques that are used to elicit responses from patients and providers alike. The results of this work are used by regulatory and reimbursement decision makers in countries throughout the world to different degrees.

This section concludes with Chapter 5, which provides an overview of statistical analysis in biomedical research. The chapter is not intended to be a review of basic biostatistics but covers some of the topics that are more important to pharmacoeconomics and health outcome research such as basic study design, source for errors in measurement, review of basic properties of probabilities, various theoretical probability distributions commonly encountered, and basic measures of risk, as well as regression analyses to adjust for differences in baseline characteristics across comparison groups.

Introduction

George E. MacKinnon III, PhD, RPh, FASHP

"Not everything that can be counted counts, and not everything that counts can be counted."

—Albert Einstein

Learning Objectives

- What is the best medication for the patient?
- What is the cheapest medication for the patient's condition?
- What is this medication going to cost the insurer?
- What amount of money will this medication/intervention save the health plan or hospital?
- What benefit is achieved or risks are incurred in providing this medication over another option?
- What is the best medication/intervention for a similar group of patients?
- Which medication should be added to the formulary, and which ones should be taken off?
- How should limited resources be used to obtain the optimal value (for patients, the health plan, providers, hospitals, and society)?

The questions posed in the Learning Objectives are not easy questions to answer but require consideration among all stakeholders. This book intends to assist individuals interested in learning about ways or tools to better address these questions by describing the tools used to assess patient-related health status and describing the analyses used to determine cost effectiveness in evaluating pharmacotherapeutic interventions to improve health. Given the finite resources and escalating costs associated with health care today, it is imperative that health care practitioners (present and future) understand the basis for decisions that impact the use of health care interventions, including diagnostics and pharmaceuticals. As Sir William Castell, former Chairman and CEO of GE Healthcare, was quoted as saying in the *Wall Street Journal*, "Healthcare needs to move from our greatest modern cost, to our greatest modern asset."[1] To do

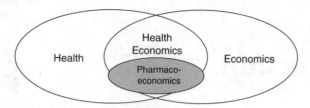

FIGURE 1-1 Health and Pharmacoeconomics.

this takes an understanding of both health care and economics. Health economics brings together these two broad disciplines. Pharmacoeconomics is a subset of health economics, as depicted in FIGURE 1-1, and has a focus on pharmaceuticals.

Since the mid-1980s, interest in the economic value and total costs associated with medication therapies has increased due to many factors. Such factors include escalating health care costs, competitive technologies and new products, increased availability of medical and prescription data, health-related quality-of-life issues, and finite resources to cover the escalating costs associated with health care.

To determine the value proposition of an intervention, this can be reduced to a simple mathematical equation:

$$\text{Value} = \frac{\text{Benefits}}{\text{Costs}}$$

While the determination of benefits and costs seems obvious, their identification can be challenging. Often it is useful to group outcomes and thus benefits into categories such as clinical (eg, physiologic, metabolic, disease prevention, morbidity, and mortality measures), humanistic (eg, quality of life, functional status, satisfaction), and economic (direct and indirect costs). Direct costs (both medical and nonmedical) are all the goods, services, and other resources that are consumed in the provision of a health intervention or in dealing with side effects. Indirect costs refer to the lost productivity suffered by the national economy as a result of an employee's absence from the workplace through illness, decreased efficiency, or premature death. FIGURES 1-2 and 1-3 depict the types of direct and indirect costs and the relative difficulty in identifying such costs.

Traditionally, product efficacy and safety have been the primary indicators for regulatory approval of drugs (eg, the Food and Drug Administration [FDA]), as well as for practitioners in assessing medication therapy outcomes. Although phase I to III studies are often well designed and carefully reviewed by the FDA for a new medication to be approved, they do have inherent limitations. Some weaknesses include limited number and range of subjects (eg, very homogeneous patients), use of surrogate end points, lack of active comparators (often compared to a placebo), relative limited time frame for the study, and absence of risk-benefit analysis. TABLE 1-1 differentiates between drug studies that focus on safety and efficacy versus clinical practice where the ultimate benefits of medications extend into overall effectiveness. For example,

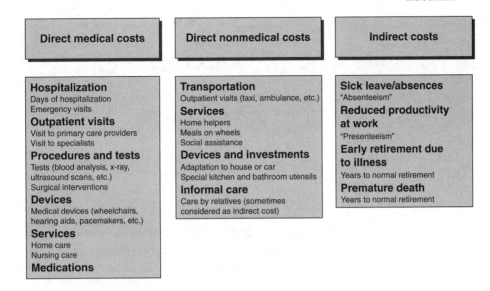

FIGURE 1-2 Measuring Direct and Indirect Medical Costs.

two medications might have an equal safety and efficacy profile, but one product is dosed four times daily and the other is dosed once daily. The once-daily medication will likely result in enhanced effectiveness in clinical practice among patients because of its convenience, fewer missed doses, and possible pharmacodynamic issues.

Due to the specific goals of randomized clinical trials (RCTs), very strict guidelines for patient eligibility are adhered to, with the result that the trials involve homogeneous patient types in small sample sizes numbering in the hundreds to thousands. As a result, the variance among patients is rather limited. Thus when products are

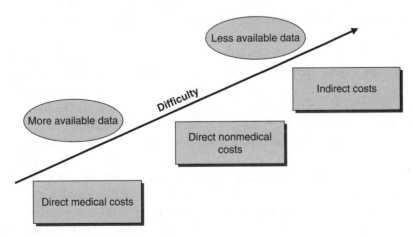

FIGURE 1-3 Difficulty in Measuring Medical Costs.

Table 1-1	From Study Drug to Medication
Drug	**Medication**
Focus: Efficacy and safety	Focus: Effectiveness
• Use in controlled clinical practice?	• Use in real-life clinical practice?
• Sample size = 100s to 1000s of patients	• Population = 10,000s to millions of patients
• Phase I-III studies	• Phase IV studies
• Homogeneous patients	• Heterogeneous patients
• Randomized clinical trials	• Postmarketing observational studies

introduced to the population at large, which can number in the tens of thousands (ie, a heterogeneous population), the outcomes of efficacy and safety may vary compared to what was observed in the RCTs. An example of the limitations of surrogate end points would be the assumptions that a reduction in blood pressure, alterations in lipids (eg, low-density lipoprotein [LDL] cholesterol reductions and high-density lipoprotein [HDL] increases), or stabilization of blood glucose (eg, hemoglobin A1c) are assumed to translate into health benefits such as reduced cardiovascular events or complications of diabetes. Lastly, there is an overall lack of an ongoing evaluation of the safety and efficacy of medications during their market life.

Unfortunately, the prescription coverage offered by many health plans is "carved out" from the overall health care benefit. As a result, the benefits (and costs) of medications may be understated or overstated. Why might this be of concern? Take for example a product (Product A) that has a drug acquisition cost of $15 a month ($0.50 a day per tablet). If this product requires a laboratory blood test every week at a cost of $30, then the actual cost of therapy (prescription and laboratory) for 1 month is $135 ($15 + $30 + $30 + $30 + $30). So although the drug acquisition cost of $15 seems reasonable, if one adds in the laboratory costs, the overall cost of therapy is greater than what one might expect. Now if a new product (Product B) is available at $4.50 per tablet or $135 per month for the prescription and does not require the same laboratory monitoring as Product A, is the new product better? To answer this question, it matters from whose perspective the question is being answered.

The pharmacy costs would increase from $180 ($15/month × 12 months) per year to $1620 ($135/month × 12 months) for a change from Product A to Product B. This increase in prescription costs is 9 times the previous cost, for an increase of 800%! Thus, the pharmacy benefit management (PBM) company may not be pleased if they have been asked to hold annual prescription cost increases to less than 5% for the health plans that have contracted with them. This $1440 increase for a patient would translate to an increase of $1.44 million when covering 1000 patient lives or of $14.4 million when covering 10,000 patient lives. Therefore, these large dollar amounts get the interest of PBMs and health care plans.

Likewise, the clinical laboratory may be disappointed in that it now loses $1440 per year in laboratory revenues (not including the costs of tests, supplies, and labor). This $1440 per patient decrease in laboratory revenues would translate to a decrease of $1.44 million per 1000 patient lives. Such an impact to the financial balance sheet would get the attention of the laboratory industry very quickly. In addition, laboratory manufacturers will incur a loss of revenue in supplies and reagents associated with the elimination of laboratory tests.

For the health plan, although the prescription costs went from $180 to $1620 (an increase of $1440), the clinical laboratory costs went from $1440 to $0 (a decrease of $1440), so the net change was $0. One pharmaceutical manufacturer loses $180 in sales annually, while another manufacturer gains $1620 in sales annually. As for the patients, they have the convenience of not having to travel to a clinical laboratory to have their blood taken weekly and do not incur the costs due to travel and nonproductivity associated with possibly missing work. The employers of the patients also may realize a benefit of increased productivity from the employee as a result of reduced absenteeism associated with the weekly laboratory tests. Note that for simplicity, these costs do not include labor or professional fees or the co-pays of the patient for either prescriptions or laboratory services. FIGURE 1-4 depicts the total costs that may be attributed to a disease or condition. Clearly, the total patient costs associated with a disease or condition are extensive and impact many areas.

Although not intended to be a pharmacy-centric textbook, pharmacists, pharmacy students, and pharmacy residents by nature of their profession are involved

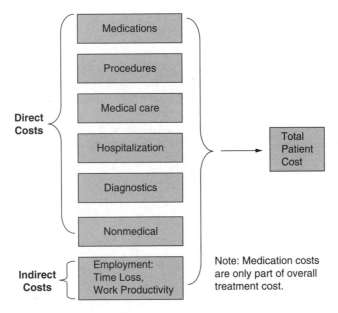

FIGURE 1-4 Total Cost Estimation of a Disease.

with pharmaceuticals and self-care products, including their procurement, distribution, monitoring, and cost-effective evaluation, more so than any other health care profession. In fact, the "Accreditation Standards and Guidelines for the Professional Program in Pharmacy Leading to the Doctor of Pharmacy Degree," as promulgated by the Accreditation Council for Pharmacy Education (ACPE), state that pharmacy graduates should be competent to "*provide population-based care*, through the ability to develop and implement population-specific, evidence-based disease management programs and protocols based upon analysis of epidemiologic and pharmacoeconomic data, medication-use criteria, medication use review, and risk-reduction strategies."[2]

However, this book has applicability to many other health care disciplines in their various levels of education and training, including but not limited to physicians, physician-assistants, nurses, therapists, and other counselors who are involved in overseeing medication use in their patients. The need for interprofessional education was made apparent in the 2003 "Health Professions Education: A Bridge to Quality" report by the Institute of Medicine (IOM)[3] as 1 of the 5 key areas elaborated upon. As recommended by the IOM, all health care professionals must be educated to deliver patient-centered care as members of an interprofessional team, *emphasizing evidence-based practice*, quality improvement approaches, and informatics. Clearly, an enhanced understanding of pharmacoeconomic principles is a step in the right direction for all health care practitioners, present and future, as we do our best to ensure optimal medication therapy outcomes for patients and society in an environment of finite resources.

■ References

1. Castell W. GE's William Castell Tells Why an Ounce of Prevention is Worth More Than a Ton of Cures. *The Wall Street Journal's Manager's Journal.* July 12, 2005: B2.
2. Accreditation Council for Pharmacy Education. Accreditation standards and guidelines for the professional program in pharmacy leading to the doctor of pharmacy degree. http://www.acpe-accredit.org/standards/default.asp. Accessed October 5, 2010.
3. Greiner AC, Knebel E, eds. *Health Professions Education: A Bridge to Quality.* Committee on the Health Profession Education Summit. Institute of Medicine. Washington, DC: National Academies Press; 2003.

Drug Development and Approval

Patricia M. Finnegan, MS
George E. MacKinnon III, PhD, RPh, FASHP

Learning Objectives

- Discuss the key drivers for the evolution of drug discovery and development processes in the United States, with respect to safety, efficacy, and effectiveness evaluation.

- Discuss the impact of the Food, Drug and Cosmetic Act, Durham-Humphrey Amendment, and Kefauver-Harris Amendments on drug regulation.

- Compare and contrast the Drug Price Competition and Patent Term Restoration Act with the Orphan Drug Act, with respect to patent protection for manufacturers.

- Identify potential concerns with the Prescription Drug User Fee Act and the integrity of the Food and Drug Administration approval process.

- Describe typical drug development activities during the pre-clinical and clinical (Phase I, II, and III) phases.

- Discuss the challenges related to FDA submissions required to conduct clinical trials and bring new drugs to market.

- Describe how the challenges associated with discovering and developing new drugs and recovering R&D costs can impact the cost of medicines.

- Become familiar with the challenges associated with the approval of biosimilars compared with generics, and the role of comparative effectiveness for biosimilars.

■ Introduction

Drug Development and Regulation at the Turn of the 20th Century

At the beginning of the 20th century, little was known about the underlying causes of most diseases, drug development was in its infancy, and there were no regulations in the United States to protect the public from exposure to dangerous and ineffective drugs. Drug makers were not required to demonstrate safety until 1938 and efficacy until 1962, before bringing a new drug to market.

Evolution of Drug Development and Approval

Forces shaping the evolution of drug development and approval processes in the United States include tragedies resulting in outcries for regulation to protect the public, the increasing cost and time to bring new therapies to patients, the escalating cost of health care, and advances in science and technology. Advances in science and technology and regulation of medical products led to the availability of many safe, effective new therapies, but not without contributing to the increasing cost and time to bring new therapies to patients and the escalating cost of health care.

Drug Development and Approval Present and Future

Drug development and approval today is a long, complex, costly process, and only a small percentage of drug candidates complete the process to become new drugs. Approval of new drugs is based on evaluation of safety and efficacy in clinical trials and on consideration of the benefits of the drug versus the risks from side effects. Clinical trials are conducted under controlled conditions and can be designed to investigate sex, ethnicity/race, and age differences; compare outcomes with other drugs and in combination with other drugs; evaluate different doses; and assess safety with long-term dosing.

In 2009, Congress passed the American Recovery and Reinvestment Act (ARRA), which provides funding to the DHHS for comparative effectiveness research (CER) and requires establishment of a Federal Coordinating Council for Comparative Effectiveness Research. Patients and clinicians often have extensive options for diagnosis, treatment, and prevention, but it is frequently unclear how to select the best option. Clinical studies for drug approval establish efficacy under controlled conditions, whereas CER evaluates effectiveness in real-world settings to provide information that clinicians and patients can use to choose the options that best fit an individual patient's needs and preferences. The Coordinating Council views comparative effectiveness as needing to complement the trend to develop personalized medicine—the ability to customize a drug and dose based on individual patient and disease characteristics.

■ Regulation

Department of Health and Human Services

The Department of Health and Human Services (DHHS) is the US government's principal agency for protecting the health of Americans and providing essential human services. The Food and Drug Administration (FDA) and National Institutes of Health (NIH) are government agencies within DHHS.

Drugs, biological products, and medical devices sold in the United States are regulated by the FDA. The FDA is also responsible for helping to speed innovations that make medicines more effective, safer, and more affordable and providing information for safe, effective use of the medicines.

FDA defines a drug as "a substance intended for use in the diagnosis, cure, mitigation, treatment, or prevention of disease, and a substance (other than food) intended to affect the structure or any function of the body."[1] Biologics are included within this definition and are generally covered by many of the same laws and regulations but are manufactured by a process using living material from humans, animals, or microorganisms. Other drugs are manufactured using chemical processes.

Several centers and offices exist under the umbrella of the FDA. The FDA's Center for Drug Evaluation and Research (CDER) regulates over-the-counter (OTC) and prescription drugs, including biological therapeutics and generic drugs. The Center for Biologics Evaluation and Research (CBER) regulates a wide range of products such as vaccines, blood and blood components, allergenics, somatic cells, gene therapy, tissues, and recombinant therapeutic proteins. The Center for Devices and Radiological Health (CDRH) regulates firms that manufacture, repackage, relabel, and/or import medical devices sold in the United States.

The FDA implements applicable laws passed by Congress by establishing regulations that become part of the Code of Federal Regulations. The FDA also issues guidance that represents the agency's current thinking on topics, but is not enforceable as regulation.

The mission of the NIH is to seek fundamental knowledge about the nature and behavior of living systems and the application of that knowledge to enhance health, lengthen life, and reduce the burdens of illness and disability.

More information about the DHHS, FDA, and NIH can be found at their respective Web sites: dhhs.gov, fda.gov, and nih.gov.

Evolution of Drug Regulation: Focus on Safety

Biologics Control Act

Following the deaths of 22 children from contaminated diphtheria antitoxin and smallpox vaccine, the Biologics Control Act of 1902 was passed to ensure the safety of serums, vaccines, and similar products. This act instituted premarket licensing for biological products and facilities, authorized inspections, and gave federal regulators the power to withhold, suspend, or revoke licenses.

Food, Drug and Cosmetic Act and Durham-Humphrey Amendment

In 1937, elixir of sulfanilamide containing the toxic solvent diethylene glycol killed 107 people, many of whom were children. The Federal Food, Drug and Cosmetic (FFDC) Act was passed in 1938, significantly expanding the scope of drug regulation. The law mandated premarket approval of drugs based on demonstration of safety by the manufacturer. Labels were to have adequate directions for safe use and were prohibited from containing false therapeutic claims. The FFDC also mandated the establishment of safe tolerances for unavoidable toxic substances and authorized inspections of factories. Soon after passage of the law, requirements for prescriptions were expanded to include potentially dangerous nonnarcotic drugs. To further define requirements for prescriptions, the Durham-Humphrey Amendment was passed in 1951 mandating the dispensing of habit-forming or potentially harmful drugs under the supervision of a health practitioner and labeled with the statement, "Caution: Federal law prohibits dispensing without prescription."

Good Manufacturing Practices

However, passage of the FFDC of 1938 was not enough to ensure the public's safety. In 1941, sulfathiazole contaminated with phenobarbital caused nearly 300 deaths and injuries. In response, changes were implemented in the regulations for manufacturing quality control. The present day version, Current Good Manufacturing Practices (CGMP), specifies minimum requirements for methods, facilities, and manufacturing controls to assure the identity, strength, and purity of drug products.

Good Laboratory Practices

In 1975, audits of contract research and industry toxicology laboratories revealed fraud, errors, inadequately trained personnel, and poor record keeping. This raised serious concerns about the validity of nonclinical safety data used to support clinical testing and marketing of drugs. As a result, Good Laboratory Practice (GLP) regulations for conducting nonclinical safety studies became effective in 1978 and, with updates, are still in effect today.

Food and Drug Administration Amendments Act

Congress passed the Food and Drug Administration Amendments Act (FDAAA) in 2007, providing resources to enhance postmarket drug safety through use of improved adverse event data collection and analysis systems, enforce requirements for postapproval studies, and report new safety concerns identified from adverse event screening. Manufacturers were required to develop risk evaluation and mitigation strategies (REMS) for drug approval and, in some cases, for drugs that were already on the market.

Evaluating Safety and Efficacy

Kefauver-Harris Drug Amendments

The drug thalidomide, approved outside of the United States and widely prescribed for pregnant women to treat morning sickness, caused serious birth defects in thousands of babies during the late 1950s and early 1960s. This led to a rapid increase in drug regulation in many countries, including the United States. In 1962, the Kefauver-Harris Drug Amendments were passed requiring drug makers to demonstrate efficacy in addition to safety for premarket approval. This law also mandated retrospective assessment of the efficacy of all drugs introduced after 1938, stricter regulation of clinical trials, and informed consent by patients participating in clinical trials. Prescription drugs were given first priority for assessment because of their greater potential for harm. There were thought to be 100,000 to 500,000 nonprescription drugs in the marketplace whose efficacy had not been evaluated. Evaluation of nonprescription drugs was started in 1972 after a study by the National Academy of Science–National Research Council suggested that only 25% were effective.

■ Sex, Age, and Racial Differences in Clinical Trials

The FDA's guidance in 1977 was to exclude women of childbearing potential from early drug studies. This was revoked in 1993, and guidance was issued for the study and evaluation of sex differences in the clinical evaluation of drugs.

In 1989, the FDA issued guidelines asking manufacturers to determine whether a drug is likely to have significant use in older people and to include older patients in clinical studies. The 1997 Food and Drug Administration Modernization Act supported accelerated approval and gave an extra period (6 months) of marketing exclusivity to manufacturers that studied a drug's effects in children. In 1998, the FDA issued the Demographic Rule requiring analysis of safety and effectiveness data by age, sex, and race. The 1998 Pediatric Rule, which was passed to require manufacturers of selected new and existing drug products to assess safety and efficacy in children, was overturned by a federal court in 2002. In 2003, the Pediatric Research Equity Act was passed, giving the FDA authority to require pediatric studies of new drugs and certain drugs already on the market.

■ Focus on Cost Control and Faster Access to New Therapies

Efforts in the United States to address the rising costs of drug development included legislation to leverage government-funded research, encourage development of therapies for rare diseases, expedite the availability of lower cost alternatives to brand name drugs, and expedite approval of new drugs. These problems were also addressed through regulatory agency and industry collaboration on ways to harmonize drug development and approval processes across certain global markets.

The Bayh-Dole Act

The Bayh-Dole Act, passed in 1980 and amended in 1984, gave universities and other nonprofit entities the opportunity to own and license the inventions they discovered through government-funded research. This was later extended to federal laboratories. Before passage of the law, the government held title to 25,000 to 30,000 inventions resulting from government-funded research but had commercially licensed only about 5%. A study published in the *New England Journal of Medicine* in 2011 concluded that public sector research inventions contributed from 9% to 21% of all New Drug Applications (NDAs) approved from 1990 through 2007.[2]

The Orphan Drug Act

The Orphan Drug Act was passed in 1983 and continues to encourage the development and marketing of drugs to treat diseases affecting fewer than 200,000 people. The law offers incentives to drug makers such as waivers of registration fees, 7 years of market exclusivity after approval, and grants for clinical trials. Nearly 350 orphan drugs have been approved since passage of the law.

Drug Price Competition and Patent Term Restoration Act

The Drug Price Competition and Patent Term Restoration Act, also called the Hatch-Waxman Amendments to the FFDC Act, was passed in 1984 allowing drug makers to request approval to market less costly generics without repeating the studies that showed the brand name drugs were safe and effective. This law also enabled manufacturers of brand name drugs to apply for up to 5 years of additional patent protection to make up for time lost while their products were going through the approval process. Generic products were estimated to account for 78% of prescriptions filled in 2010, up from 49% in 2000.[3]

Prescription Drug User Fee Act

Pressures from the public, special interest groups, and pharmaceutical manufacturers led to passage of the Prescription Drug User Fee Act (PDUFA) in 1992, which authorized collection of fees from pharmaceutical manufacturers for regulatory submissions. In essence, companies now pay a fee (originally about half a million dollars per review) for a new molecular entity (NME) and impose deadlines for completion of these drug reviews by the FDA. The deadlines vary for priority and standard NME drug reviews, presently at 6 months for priority reviews and 10 months for standard reviews. PDUFA and associated fees did have an impact, as review times went from 33 months to 19 months between 1991 and 2001. The 2010 fee for an application requiring clinical data was $1,405,500.[4] PDUFA has been reauthorized about every 5 years and most recently in 2008. Most notably, up until 2008, the fees collected could not be used for postmarket safety reviews by the FDA, only for approvals. Presently, fees account for about 50% of the budget for the center that reviews NDAs.

International Conference on Harmonization

Differences in marketing requirements often meant that time-consuming, costly studies had to be repeated and documents rewritten to bring medicines into other countries. In 1990, the International Conference on Harmonization (ICH) was formed with representatives from regulatory agencies and pharmaceutical industry associations in Europe, Japan, and the United States. ICH developed best practice guidance for drug development activities impacting safety, quality, and efficacy, such as nonclinical safety testing, clinical trials, setting manufacturing specifications, performing quality control testing, determining storage conditions and shelf life, and quality risk management.

The ICH developed a standard format called the Common Technical Document (CTD) for assembling the quality, safety, and efficacy information for market application. Use of the CTD has eliminated the need to reformat documents for submission to different ICH regulatory authorities, simplified the review process for regulatory agencies, and facilitated implementation of electronic regulatory submissions. Prior to implementation of the CTD and electronic submissions, regulatory agencies received truckloads of paper documents, varying in format from company to company, to review for approval of new drugs. The ICH also developed standardized medical terminology (Medical Dictionary for Regulatory Activities), for use in applying for market authorization and monitoring the safety of medical products. The ICH maintains a Web site (www .ich.org), where information about the group's history and current activities is available.

■ Drug Discovery, Development, and Approval

Overview

As depicted in FIGURE 2-1, the process of discovering, developing, and obtaining approval to bring a new medicine to patients has been estimated to take an average of 10 to 15 years and cost from $1.2 to $1.3 billion. As few as 1 in 5000 to 10,000 new molecular entities created during the discovery phase may lead to approval of a new drug.[3]

A potential new drug can fail at any stage, including at the end of phase III clinical testing after a considerable investment in time and resources. Only about 9% of drugs entering phase I reach the market.[5] Failure is often due to difficulties in predicting efficacy and safety in nonclinical testing and early in clinical trials.

Even after a new drug is approved, there is no guarantee that the discovery, development, and launch costs will be recovered. Only 2 of 10 drugs brought to market are

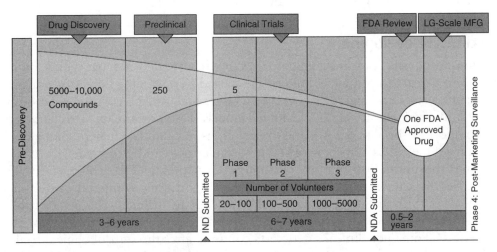

FIGURE 2-1 Drug development process.

Source: Reprinted with permission from PhRMA Brochure, Drug discovery and development, copyright 2007.

estimated to return revenues that match or exceed research and development costs.[3] Market exclusivity is limited by the patent life remaining when a drug is approved, and patents are often contested by other drug makers, particularly if the drug is widely used. Competitive products are often approved soon after launch. New side effects observed after a drug is widely prescribed or during postmarket clinical trials can limit its use or cause it to be withdrawn from the market. New products are not always well accepted by patients and health care providers. A new drug may not achieve the expected improvements in health outcomes because of patient nonadherence to therapy. Despite harmonization of technical requirements for marketing approval among the ICH member countries, approval in one country does not guarantee approval in others. The cost of manufacturing a drug and maintaining it on the market can be high compared to the price that can be charged and the sales volume.

Drug Discovery

Drug discovery starts with an unmet medical need and knowledge from basic research about a disease process that suggests a target that a drug can act on to alter the progress of the disease. During the discovery stage, ideas about molecular structures that might be effective in acting on the target are developed and evaluated. Potential drugs are made in small amounts using chemical synthesis or biological systems and screened for activity and toxicity. Substances that show promise, or lead compounds, are modified and evaluated for improvements in activity and reduction of toxicity. The desired attributes, or target candidate profile, guide the selection and optimization of leads. A new drug should offer significant improvements over the best currently available therapy and what is known about new therapies currently under development. However, one of the challenges during drug discovery is that screening methods often have a limited capacity for predicting outcomes in humans.

Preclinical Development

The most promising, or lead, candidates advance to a preclinical stage, which can take from 3 to 6 years to complete. Studies are started to determine how to produce the active pharmaceutical ingredient (API) on a larger scale and prepare formulations for safety studies in laboratory tests and animal models. Tests are developed to characterize the composition of both the API and formulations. A candidate may be eliminated at this stage if the API is not stable or stable formulations cannot be made.

The adsorption, distribution, metabolism, excretion, and toxicologic (ADMET) properties are studied in living cells and animals and using computational models. The goals of the nonclinical safety evaluation generally include a characterization of toxic effects with respect to target organs and dose dependence and reversibility of side effects. Some nonclinical safety tests continue after the start of clinical trials to determine whether there are any long-term adverse effects in animals that might appear in humans. Nonclinical safety studies performed to support clinical testing and marketing of new drugs must comply with GLPs for Nonclinical Laboratory Studies regulations.

Nonclinical ADMET studies are used to estimate an initial safe starting dose and dose range for clinical studies and to identify parameters to monitor for potential adverse effects in humans. Dosage form development studies explore different packaging and formulations (eg, pill, inhaler, injection). Scale-up of API and dosage form preparation to support manufacture of clinical supplies is continued. Clinical plans and requirements for supplies of the active ingredient and dosage form(s) for use in the clinical studies are developed. All clinical trial plans must be reviewed and approved by the institutional review board (IRB) at the institutions where the trials will take place (eg, hospitals, medical offices).

Investigational New Drug Application

Before clinical trials begin, an Investigational New Drug Application (INDA) is filed with the FDA. The application includes preclinical safety data, the drug candidate's chemical structure, proposed mechanism of action, listing of any side effects, and manufacturing information for both the API and dosage form. The INDA also includes a detailed clinical trial plan that outlines how, where, and by whom the studies will be performed. The FDA has only 30 days to review the INDA. Unless the FDA orders a "clinical hold," the clinical trial can be started at the end of the 30-day review period.

Clinical Studies

Clinical studies must be conducted in compliance with Good Clinical Practice (GCP) regulations. GCP is a standard for the design, conduct, performance, monitoring, auditing, recording, analysis, and reporting of clinical trials or studies. The FDA requires that all drugs and devices undergoing clinical trials in humans must be registered on the Clinical Trials Database maintained by the agency (www.clinicaltrials.gov). In addition to a registry of clinical trials that are recruiting or accepting patients, active and not recruiting, or complete, it contains the links to relevant information, including FDA advisory committee summary documents related to the drug or device. At present, the registry has over 86,000 clinical trials registered and the results of over 1500 studies posted.

The emphasis in phase I studies is on safety. Studies are conducted with limited dosing and a small number of volunteers, usually about 20 to 80. Information about how the drug is absorbed, metabolized, and excreted in humans may also be obtained for comparison with the nonclinical data.

Phase II studies begin if no unacceptable toxicity is observed during phase I. The goal of phase II is to obtain preliminary data on whether the drug is effective in treating the disease in humans. In controlled trials, patients receiving the drug are compared with homogenous patient types receiving a different treatment such as an inactive substance (ie, placebo) or a different drug. Safety also continues to be evaluated, and short-term side effects are studied. ADMET data may also be obtained during this phase. The number of subjects in phase II studies ranges from a few dozen to about

300. At the end of phase II, both the FDA and sponsors come to an agreement on how the large-scale studies in phase III should be conducted. Data from the phase II studies are used to determine the dosages to study in phase III.

Phase III studies begin if there is evidence of efficacy and no safety concerns from phase II. Phase III studies gather more information about safety and efficacy of the drug in diverse populations at different dosages and in combination with other drugs. The studies have to be large enough to support statistically significant conclusions about the safety and efficacy of the drug. The number of subjects can range from several hundred to 5000. Statisticians and others monitor data as they become available throughout the study. The FDA or the sponsor can stop the trial at any time if problems arise. In some cases, a study may be stopped because the drug candidate is performing so well that it would be unethical to withhold it from the patients receiving a placebo or another drug. The company sponsoring the research must provide regular comprehensive reports to the FDA and the IRB on the progress of clinical trials.

Application for Approval of a New Drug

Once all three phases of the clinical trials are complete, the sponsor analyzes all of the data to determine whether the experimental medicine is both safe and effective. The sponsor may decide not proceed with a market application if the drug fails to offer a significant improvement over existing therapies, or because of new knowledge about the disease process. Sponsors often meet with the FDA at the end of phase III and just before submission of an application for approval. An NDA is submitted for a drug with a chemically synthesized API, and a Biological License Application (BLA) is submitted for a drug manufactured using biological systems.

FDA Review and Approval

NDAs are typically 100,000 pages or longer and contain information about nonclinical testing, clinical trials, manufacturing details, and proposed labeling. The FDA has implemented the Electronic Submission Gateway, allowing a submission to be sent electronically much like an e-mail. FDA scientists review the information in the application to determine whether the medicine is safe and effective and the manufacturing meets quality requirements. There is risk of an adverse reaction with any drug, and consideration of whether the benefits outweigh the risks is part of the review process. The sponsor can request a priority review for a drug that appears to offer an advance over available therapy or an orphan drug review for a product that treats a rare disease affecting fewer than 200,000 Americans. Other applications are given a standard review.

The FDA sometimes seeks additional opinions by convening an advisory committee meeting with a panel of experts appointed by the FDA. The advisory committee evaluates data presented by company representatives and FDA reviewers, and votes on whether the application should be approved and under what conditions. The FDA is not required to follow the recommendations of the advisory committee, but often does.

Before making a decision for approval, the FDA may conduct a preapproval inspection of the proposed manufacturing facilities and request additional information from the sponsor. Approval is sometimes granted with conditions that must be met after initial marketing, such as conducting additional clinical studies to evaluate risks and benefits in a different population or conducting special monitoring in a high-risk population.

Postapproval Activities

Drug makers are required to report adverse drug reactions at quarterly intervals for the first 3 years after approval, including a special report for any serious and unexpected adverse reactions. Postmarketing surveillance is important, because phase III studies might not uncover every adverse reaction that could be observed once a drug is widely prescribed in the heterogeneous population at large. The FDA has set up a medical reporting program called MedWatch to track serious adverse events.

Generic Drugs

A generic drug is a copy of an off-patent innovator's drug made by a chemical process. Passage of the Hatch-Waxman Amendments to the FFDC Act in 1984 allowed manufacturers of generic drugs to rely on the findings of safety and efficacy of the previously approved drug, called the reference listed drug (RLD), for approval. Thus generic companies do not have to repeat expensive nonclinical and clinical trials.

Requirements for a generic drug compared with the RLD include:

- Same active ingredient(s)
- Same route of administration
- Same dosage form
- Same strength
- Same conditions of use

Approval for a generic drug is requested using an Abbreviated New Drug Application (ANDA). The generic sponsor must perform studies to show bioequivalence to the RLD and provide manufacturing information. Bioequivalence is defined as pharmaceutical equivalents whose rate and extent of absorption are not statistically different when administered to patients or subjects at the same molar dose under similar experimental conditions. An ANDA may be submitted before expiry of the innovator's patent, allowing the generic to be approved and marketed very rapidly after expiry of the innovator's patent.

The "Orange Book" contains RLDs/brand name drugs identified by the FDA for generic companies to compare with their proposed products as well as patent expiration dates. The therapeutic equivalence codes described in the Orange Book are "A," which indicates substitutable, and "B," which indicates inequivalent, not substitutable. All FDA-approved drug products listed include NDAs, ANDAs, and OTCs. OTCs are described in a following section.

Biosimilars

The active ingredients in drugs made by chemical processes are typically small molecules containing 20 to 100 atoms. These molecules can be well-characterized, purified, and analyzed with routine laboratory tests. Relatively speaking, small molecules are easy to produce and manufacture.

In contrast, the active ingredients in biologics are much larger molecules. Small biologics, such as hormones, contain 200 to 3000 atoms, and large biologics, such as antibodies, contain 5000 to 50,000 atoms.

Biologics are typically produced using living cell lines developed by the innovator and tend to be diverse mixtures of molecules that differ very slightly from one another. Biologics replicate the natural enzymes, antibodies, or hormones found in our bodies. Classes of biologics include hormones, vaccines, recombinant DNA proteins, monoclonal antibodies, enzymes, and immunomodulators.

Unlike drug products produced by chemical processes, the size and complexity of biologics make them very difficult to characterize. When a biologic is produced with cell lines developed by another manufacturer, it may be similar but will probably not be identical to the innovator's product. By nature of the production involved to create biologics, they are often not very stable, require refrigeration or freezing for storage, are commonly produced as injectables, and are costly (eg, some doses are in the thousands of dollars).

Differences in protein glycosylation can result in immunogenicity, a significant concern for biosimilars. Glycosylation is important in that it serves as tags that aid recognition of target receptors and modulates protein folding into three-dimensional tertiary and quaternary structures, thereby conferring stability to the protein. Differences in glycosylation can affect several key parameters including half-life, distribution, solubility, stability, target affinity, receptor binding, and immunogenicity.

Biosimilars are approved on the basis that they are equal to the reference biologic in terms of both efficacy and safety. Biosimilars are unique products but not generic versions of the innovator biologic and cannot be substituted for brand name biologics without prescriber approval.

The Patient Protection and Affordable Care (PPAC) Act, also called the Biologics Price Competition and Innovation (BPCI) Act, was signed into law on March 23, 2010, to create an abbreviated approval pathway for biological products that are demonstrated to be highly similar (biosimilar) to or interchangeable with an FDA-approved biological product. The FDA is expected to announce plans for implementation of the law in 2011.

Over-the-Counter Drugs

The FDA requires OTC drugs to be safe and effective for use by the general public without a doctor's prescription. OTCs must meet the same standards for safety and effectiveness as prescription drugs. OTCs manufactured and labeled in accordance with monographs published in the Code of Federal Regulations (21 CFR parts 331–358) do not require premarket approval. All other OTC products require premarket approval through submission of an NDA or ANDA. Consumers must be able to use the drug appropriately and safely, and this can be assessed with label comprehension and actual-use studies. Drugs initially approved as prescription only may be approved later as OTCs. Some examples are Advil, Claritin, and Zantac.

Drug Development and Approval in the Future

Drug development and approval processes in the United States will continue to be shaped by desires for regulation to protect the public, the increasing cost and time to bring new therapies to patients, the escalating cost of health care, and advances in science and technology. There are no quick fixes for the problems of increasing cost and time to bring new products to market and the escalating cost of health care; however, there are a number of ongoing initiatives that offer opportunities for improvement. Funding for some of these efforts may be limited because of the US budget deficit.

Despite efforts to bring new therapies to patients faster, applications and approvals for new molecular entities (NMEs), where NME applications include both NDAs and BLAs, have failed to show any real growth over the last 4 years, as shown in FIGURES 2-2 and 2-3.

Increased globalization of medical products manufacturing presents new challenges for regulators. In the wake of 2008 recalls of heparin found to contain contaminated API manufactured in China, the FDA announced plans to boost inspection of overseas plants manufacturing pharmaceuticals distributed in the United States.

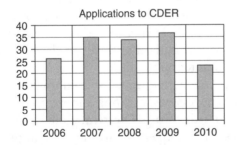

Calendar Year	Applications Filed
2006	26
2007	35
2008	34
2009	37
2010	23

NME applications to CDER are not increasing. If the number of applications does not increase, CDER does not expect to see much of a year-to-year increase in approvals.

FIGURE 2-2 NME applications to Center for Drug Evaluation and Research for 2006 to 2010. Applications for NMEs were filed under NDAs and original BLAs.

Source: Reprinted from US Food and Drug Administration New molecular entity 2010 statistics, Food and Drug Administration Web site. http://www.fda.gov/downloads/Drugs/DevelopmentApprovalProcess/HowDrugsareDevelopedandApproved/DrugandBiologicApprovalReports/UCM242695.pdf. Accessed June 1, 2011.

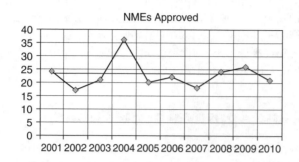

Calendar Year	NMEs Approved
2001	24
2002	17
2003	21
2004	36
2005	20
2006	22
2007	18
2008	24
2009	26
2010	21

Since 2001 CDER has averaged slightly fewer than 23 NME approvals per year (22.9), similar to the 21 approved in 2010.

FIGURE 2-3 Ten-year average NME approvals by Center for Drug Evaluation and Research (CDER) per year. 2004–2010 represents applications for NMEs filed under NDAs and therapeutic biologics file under BLAs; 2001–2003 represents NMEs but not therapeutic biologics.

Source: Reprinted from US Food and Drug Administration. New molecular entity 2010 statistics, Food and Drug Administration Web site. http://www.fda.gov/downloads/Drugs/DevelopmentApprovalProcess/HowDrugsareDevelopedandApproved/DrugandBiologicApprovalReports/UCM242695.pdf. Accessed June 1, 2011.

CER offers the opportunity to improve health outcomes and reduce the cost of health care through the selection of health care options that provide the greatest benefit at the lowest cost. The ARRA provided funding for CER to "accelerate the development and dissemination of research assessing the comparative effectiveness of health care treatments and strategies, through efforts that: (1) conduct, support, or synthesize research that compares the clinical outcomes, effectiveness, and appropriateness of items, services, and procedures that are used to prevent, diagnose, or treat diseases, disorders, and other health conditions; and (2) encourage the development and use of clinical registries, clinical data networks, and other forms of electronic health data that can be used to generate or obtain outcomes data."

The Patent Reform Act of 2011, if enacted, may speed innovation and protect inventors by shortening times for patent reviews, creating a more predictable system, and moving from a first-to-invent to a first-to-file system, as used by competitors abroad. The bill may also lower fees for "small entity inventors" and provide the US Patent and Trademark Office with resources to reduce the backlog of patent applications, which was 708,535 at the end of 2010.

The FDA's Critical Path Initiative, launched in 2004, is continuing efforts to improve the way drugs, biological products, and medical devices are developed, evaluated, and manufactured. On February 24, 2010, the FDA announced the Advancing Regulatory Science Initiative in collaboration with the NIH to speed the translation of research into medical products and therapies. The FDA defines regulatory science as "the science of developing new tools, standards and approaches to assess the safety, efficacy, quality and performance of FDA-regulated products."[6]

The NIH has proposed the formation of a new center to accelerate the development and delivery of new, more effective therapeutics. The center would develop and offer innovative services and expertise in moving promising products through the development pipeline, as well as develop novel approaches to therapeutics development, stimulate new avenues for basic scientific discovery, and complement the strengths of existing NIH research activities.

The ICH is continuing work on the global front to prevent duplication of clinical trials, minimize the use of animal testing, streamline the regulatory assessment process for NDAs, and reduce the development times and resources needed for drug development.

■ Summary

Many hurdles have been overcome since the turn of the 20th century to bring health care from where it was then to where it is today. In 2007, Americans spent $286.5 billion on prescriptions, of which $40.3 billion was on biologics; thus, the impact of biologics and subsequent biosimilars will be profound and have repercussions for all stakeholders involved with their use in health care. The challenge for the 21st century will be to find ways to bring innovative, effective therapies to patients faster, without sacrificing quality and safety, to improve health outcomes, and at the same time to lower health care costs.

■ References

1. Drugs@FDA Glossary of Terms Page, Food and Drug Administration Web site. http://www.fda.gov/Drugs/informationondrugs/ucm079436.htm. Accessed June 1, 2011

2. Stevens A, Jensen J, Wyller K, et al. The role of public-sector research in the discovery of drugs and vaccines. *N Engl J Med*. 2011;364(6):540.

3. Industry Profile 2011 Key Facts page. Pharmaceutical Research and Manufacturers of America Web Site. http://www.phrma.org/sites/default/files/159/phrma_profile_2011_final.pdf. Accessed June 2, 2011.

4. Notices. Federal Register, Vol. 74, No. 206, October 27, 2009. http://edocket.access.gpo.gov/2009/pdf/E9-25804.pdf. Accessed May 12, 2011.

5. US Food and Drug Administration. Innovation/stagnation: challenge and opportunity on the critical path to new medical products. http://nipte.org/docs/Critical_Path.pdf. Accessed May 12, 2011.

6. US Food and Drug Administration. Science and research special topics. http://www.fda.gov/ScienceResearch/SpecialTopics/default.htm. Accessed May 12, 2011.

■ Additional Resources

International Conference on Harmonization. Homepage. http://www.ich.org. Accessed May 12, 2011.

International Conference on Harmonization. The value and benefits of ICH to drug regulatory authorities. http://www.ich.org/ichnews/publications/browse/article/the-value-and-benefits-of-ich-to-drug-regulatory-authorities.html. Accessed May 12, 2011.

National Institutes of Health. Homepage. http://nih.gov/. Accessed May 12, 2011.

PhRMA. Drug discovery and development. http://www.phrma.org/research/drug-discovery-development. Accessed May 12, 2011.

PhRMA. Homepage. http://www.phrma.org/. Accessed May 12, 2011.

US Department of Health and Human Services. Homepage. http://www.hhs.gov/. Accessed May 12, 2011.

US Department of Health and Human Services. Federal Coordinating Council for Comparative Effectiveness Research Report to the President and Congress, June 30, 2009. http://www.hhs.gov/recovery/programs/cer/cerannualrpt.pdf. Accessed May 12, 2011.

US Food and Drug Administration. Advancing regulatory science for public health. http://www.fda.gov/downloads/ScienceResearch/SpecialTopics/RegulatoryScience/UCM228444.pdf. Accessed May 12, 2011.

US Food and Drug Administration. A history of the FDA and drug regulation in the United States. http://www.fda.gov/downloads/Drugs/ResourcesForYou/Consumers/BuyingUsingMedicineSafely/UnderstandingOver-the-CounterMedicines/UCM093550.pdf. Accessed May 12, 2011.

US Food and Drug Administration. Homepage. http://www.fda.gov. Accessed May 12, 2011.

US Patent and Trade Mark Office. Homepage. http://www.uspto.gov/. Accessed May 12, 2011.

Measuring Health Status and Health-Related Quality-of-Life

Nalin Payakachat, BPharm, MSc, PhD
Matthew M. Murawski, BPharm, PhD

Learning Objectives

- Define health status, health-related quality-of-life (HRQL), and the related terms quality of life, patient-reported outcomes, quality-adjusted life-year, and disability-adjusted life-year.

- Describe the importance and purposes of measuring health status and HRQL.

- Identify essential domains of HRQL measures.

- Recall the process of HRQL instrument development.

- Explain the psychometric properties of HRQL instruments and why they are important.

- Illustrate how to measure health status and HRQL.

■ Introduction

With health care costs sky-rocketing, health decision makers, including medical professionals, policy makers, and even patients, are under tremendous pressure to develop public policy and make better-informed decisions to more efficiently allocate scarce health care resources. Direct health care costs such as hospital expenditures, physician visits, and pharmacy charges can be measured and determined. Less tangible and thus more challenging to assess are the indirect costs of health care, such as lost productivity from illness or health consequences from diseases or treatments themselves. Health care's own success has meant that the majority of treatment efforts are aimed at dealing with slowly progressive, chronic diseases. In such an environment, where curing disease is rarely possible, directly quantifying a patient's health status and incorporating it into treatment evaluation alongside cost-effectiveness analysis has approached physiologic status evaluation in importance. Ideally, the goal of providing health care is to improve or at least maintain general health and the overall functional capacity of patients.

To improve a patient's health, treatment requires a specific knowledge of current levels of health, which can be compared to past and future states of health. Such measurement is a fundamental scientific activity in which researchers acquire knowledge about people, objects, phenomena, and processes by observing and quantifying them. Measuring health outcomes is not merely an aspirational objective for delivering health care; it is now a key element of clinical practice, providing crucial information about how patients respond to treatments/interventions. Likewise, health care outcomes are an important consideration for policy makers.[1]

The World Health Organization (WHO) describes health as "a state of complete physical, mental, and social well-being and not merely the absence of disease or infirmity."[2] This concept guides how health care researchers develop instruments or methods to measure health. Health is recognized as a multidimensional concept, because any single health perspective is uncertain and dissimilar. Illness can impact health in many different ways. Historically, health care mainly focused on physiologic and anatomic changes from diseases or conditions that were usually measured by physicians and surrogate outcomes (eg, blood glucose for diabetes, blood pressure for hypertension). Clinical, physiologic, and surrogate outcomes are not sufficient to describe or evaluate health consequences and may not directly correspond to health status. Yet often, the changes in patients' overall health and quality of being were overlooked. Over the past 3 decades, health status and quality-of-life measures have begun to offer information obtained directly from patients regarding the effects of treatment, both favorable and unfavorable.

The revolution in thinking has been to systematically ask patients to report how they feel in response to treatment and document their responses in an ongoing manner, when treating patients with chronic conditions. Patient-reported outcomes, combined with traditional clinical data, are playing an increasing role in the decision-making process and are distinct from traditional clinical measures. Today, health care researchers are increasingly interested in identifying how to effectively evaluate patient-reported outcomes and how to include them in economic evaluation of treatment.

■ Measurement of Health

To better understand the measurement of health, defining several terms is necessary. *Health status* is a patient's current health state, including both physical and mental wellness, as affected by any underlying diseases or medical conditions. *Quality of life (QOL)* is a broad-ranging concept that is defined by the WHO as "an individual's perception of their position in life in the context of the culture and value systems in which they live and in relation to their goals, expectations, standards, and concerns."[3] This definition implies a subjective evaluation that is embedded in a patient's particular cultural, social, and personal environment. In contrast, *health-related quality-of-life (HRQL)* is specific to health; it is restricted to only those aspects of life that may change due to illness.

The terms QOL and HRQL sometimes appear interchangeably in health care research literature, although they are conceptually distinct. Because the definitions of both QOL and HRQL focus on respondents' perceived quality of life, they are not expected to reflect the details of symptoms, diseases, or conditions, but rather the impact of the disease and health interventions on the patients' quality of life—the experience of illness. As such, QOL and HRQL cannot be equated simply with "health status," which requires a clinician's input.

It is the nature of HRQL or health states to change over time. Change can either reflect frank physical change or psychological factors that allow the patient to perceive the illness experience differently. Physical changes include the acquisition of new skills to help cope with a disability. Psychological adaptations refer to changes in people's perceptions that occur over time in response to their health state. Because cultural, social, and even spiritual factors may influence patient perception, predicting the HRQL of a specific individual is nearly impossible.

Any one person's evaluation of their well-being is dependent on a highly individualistic combination of attributes and how those attributes are weighted, in a manner that is highly unlikely to apply to another individual. In some sense, every person has their own definition of HRQL. This makes HRQL difficult to define. Because it is an intangible construct, not subject to direct measurement, it is difficult to quantify in a manner that is acceptable to all stakeholders (eg, patients, health care practitioners, payors). Current conceptualizations of HRQL include the ability to engage in everyday activities plus general health and well-being, psychological and emotional states, and sometimes social and economic stress.

Patient-reported outcomes (PROs) is a term that has gained prominence recently in the health care industry, after the US Food and Drug Administration (FDA) launched a draft guidance on PRO measures to support labeling claims in 2006.[4] PRO refers to any aspect of a patient's health status that comes directly from the patient without any interpretation by anyone else and includes symptoms, HRQL aspects, treatment adherence, and treatment satisfaction. PROs have grown in importance, especially for diseases, conditions, or treatment effects that are known only to the patient, such as pain intensity or pain relief, for which no observable or surrogate measures exist.

Clinicians and patients may benefit from HRQL or PRO measures in at least two ways: (1) using evidence to inform the decision-making authorities regarding alternative treatments, and (2) gathering needed data about patients' functioning and well-being to alert clinicians to problems that require intervention and ultimately improve patient outcomes.[5] Policy makers may also use PRO evidence and incorporate it into the decision-making process. HRQL measures are commonly included in many randomized controlled trials (RCTs) as either primary or secondary end points to evaluate patients' optimal medical management. More discussion of RCTs is provided in Chapter 6.

Several popular metrics are used when incorporating HRQL into economic analysis. *Quality-adjusted life-years* (QALYs) are the most popular HRQL metric and can be used in cost-effectiveness analysis. QALYs represent the value of a given health state weighted by duration. First, for a given intervention, a series of quality-weighted health states or utility values are determined for the health states experienced during that intervention (from death = 0; to perfect health = 1).[6] Once the quality weights are obtained for each state, they are multiplied by the time spent in the state. These products are added together to obtain the total number of QALYs.

Alternatives to QALYs include health-years equivalents (HYEs),[7] saved young life equivalents,[8] and disability-adjusted life-years (DALYs).[9] HYEs avoid certain restrictive assumptions about preferences by permitting the rate of trade-off between life-years and quality-of-life to depend on the life span. However, HYEs do not offer a practical solution to the problem of assigning utilities to health profiles for various qualities of life because they have to be calculated for every possible duration of time in the health state. DALYs were developed as the measurement unit for the Global Burden of Disease study. They have been used widely in a large group of international health interventions in which health outcomes are reported as cost per DALY. Whereas QALY weights are based on social preferences, DALY weights also incorporate age adjustments, based implicitly on economic productivity. However, questions remain about the equity and ethics of the age weightings (eg, DALYs are based on Japanese life tables).[10] More details on QOL metrics, uses in economic analysis, and their limitations[11] can be found in Chapters 3 and 4.

Seeking information from patients is not a new concept. Physicians have traditionally used informal discussion to inform their clinical judgments. However, a formal, systematic assessment such as a structured interview or standardized questionnaire provides more reliable and consistent information than an informal interview. It can minimize measurement error and ensure consistency. Health can be measured through clinical, physiologic, and surrogate outcomes as well as HRQL aspects. However, as already discussed, for certain disease states or interventions, incorporation of the patient's perspective offers unique advantages.

The HRQL construct, as a consequence of illness, is typically measured on five dimensions: physical functioning, role and social functioning, psychological functioning, general health perceptions, and other functions. Other functions may be included when assessing the treatment of a specific disease or condition, such as measures of vision functioning when assessing treatment of glaucoma. The HRQL construct cannot be directly measured by any traditional means. Health constructs relate to how patients feel or function with respect to their health.

Some constructs are directly observable or can be verified, such as walking ability; others are unobservable, such as depression. Most researchers would agree that depression is not equivalent to the behaviors they observe, but underlies it. Unobservable phenomena have to be inferred through other variables; for this reason, they are called "latent variables." The term *latent variable* refers to the underlying construct that a measurement instrument attempts to quantify. (*Note:* The term *instrument* in this chapter refers to a set of question items in an HRQL questionnaire survey, which comes along with its instructions, administration protocol, scoring guidelines, interpretation of results, and user manual.) The instrument may be made up of measures of a set of variables, or questions that are used to determine or define a construct. Sometimes, the process of measurement can reduce the dimensionality of the data. Constructs are a staple of psychological and economic research. For example, "intelligence" can be measured using IQ test questions (eg, psychology), and "customer satisfaction" can be measured through a series of questions (eg, marketing).

A conceptual model (FIGURE 3-1) shows the relationship between individual outcomes and HRQL. The model begins with an illness; it has a direct impact on 5 dimensions that will determine the HRQL construct. Clinical and surrogate outcomes show how the disease causes physiologic and anatomic changes. However, these physical changes usually do not correlate well with HRQL measures. For example, forced expiratory volume in 1 second, carbon monoxide lung diffusion capacity, and exercise test performance correlated poorly with HRQL measures in candidates for lung resection with lung cancer.[12]

Ecologic, health care, and individual characteristics are independent factors that can also influence HRQL. Ecologic characteristics include a patient's family, community, and environment. Health care characteristics include the type of health care system, availability of providers, the level of managed care penetration, insurance market competition, and the like. Individual characteristics refer to demographics and socioeconomic status. These factors can also influence each other. Physical, psychological, and role and

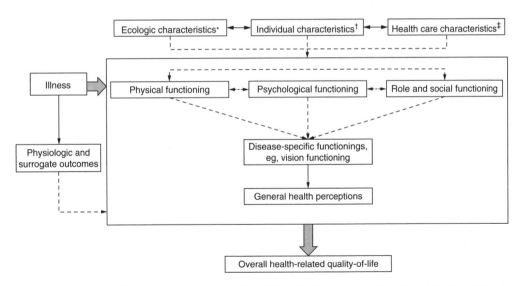

FIGURE 3-1 Relationship among measures of individual outcomes in a health-related quality-of-life conceptual model.

*Ecologic characteristics refer to human ecology such as family, community, and environment that influence human behaviors. †Individual characteristics refer to demographic and socioeconomic characteristics such as age, sex, race/ethnicity, household income, and educational level. ‡Health care characteristics refer to type of health care system, availability of health care providers, managed care penetration, and so on. A solid line refers to direct effect, whereas a dashed line refers to indirect effect.

social functioning indirectly affect each other. For example, older adults who received treatment for depression reported improvement in physical function.[13]

A disease-specific functioning can either be affected directly by the illness itself or indirectly be impacted by any changes in physical, psychological, or role and social functioning. For example, individuals with low vision functioning experienced emotional distress and significant reductions in HRQL, outcomes that were comparable to people with chronic illnesses.[14] Visual acuity was also related to one's ability to carry out daily activities. Similarly, psychological and role and social functioning, which related to vision, can be influenced by either decreased physical or disease-specific functioning. Finally, evidence from recent publications shows that patients suffering from age-related macular degeneration nonetheless sometimes reported full health.[15,16] Therefore, vision functioning is believed to be separate from physical, psychological, and role and social functioning and may not be well captured by generic HRQL instruments.[16,17] Readers will learn more about generic and disease-specific QOL instruments in Chapter 4.

■ HRQL Instrument Development

HRQL measurement instruments are collections of systematically developed questions (items) intended to quantify levels of theoretical variables not readily observable by direct means. Although more haphazard approaches sometimes appear in the literature, these approaches lead to the risk of yielding inaccurate data, the costs of which may be greater than any benefits attained.[18] A high level of measurement error imposes an absolute limit on the validity of any conclusions reached, precluding the use of the results to inform decision making. Therefore, the use of credible instruments in HRQL outcomes research is crucial.

However, developing a credible HRQL instrument entails commitment of considerable time, money, and effort. In contrast, there are more than 2000 PubMed citations for PRO instrument development articles since 1995,[19] and at least 656 with more than 1000 translations are available for PRO and HRQL instruments.[20] Health care researchers must first determine whether there is any available existing instrument that they can possibly use in the context of their research questions and in their population of interest. Selection of an available instrument for these "naïve" applications can be difficult.[21] If no suitable instrument exists, developing a specific-purpose measurement instrument may be the only remaining option.

Theory can play an important role in how instrument developers conceptualize their measurement problems. Measuring intangible phenomena derived from multiple, evolving theories poses a clear challenge to developers. The conceptual framework of an instrument is the first place to start to understand the intent of the developer so that researchers can determine whether the instrument can be adapted to or adopted for their research. Psychometric properties including reliability and validity are the next important aspect of HRQL instruments that researchers should review. Again, if there are no instruments that meet the research requirements, researchers may consider developing a new instrument. The FDA draft guidance on PRO instrument development includes four steps: (1) identify the concepts and develop a conceptual framework, (2) create an instrument, (3) assess the measurement properties, and (4) modify the instrument (FIGURE 3-2).[4]

A conceptual framework is necessary to guide a multidimensional measurement model that evaluates functioning across the principal domains mentioned earlier. It also informs selection of constructs, item development, and psychometric testing.[19] Developers must clearly identify concepts and domains that are appropriate and important to patients. Specifying a target population is a critical step for new instrument development because HRQL measures are designed to reflect patients' perception of their specific conditions. Obtaining information directly from patients would be an ideal goal. In situations where patients are too young or too old, too ill, or cognitively impaired, information obtained from a proxy may be used. To create domains and generate questions (item generation) in each HRQL domain, developers should indicate which techniques they used to evaluate an instrument's content and construct validity.

The first step in identifying what information is known about the condition of interest is the literature review. Following that, face-to-face patient interviews or focus-group

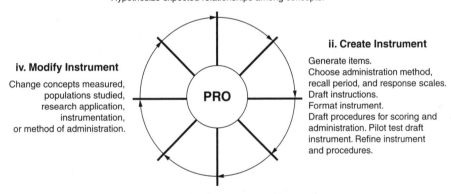

i. Idenify Concepts and Develop Conceptual Framework

Identify concepts and domains that are important to patients.
Determine intended population and research application.
Hypothesize expected relationships among concepts.

ii. Create Instrument

Generate items.
Choose administration method, recall period, and response scales.
Draft instructions.
Format instrument.
Draft procedures for scoring and administration. Pilot test draft instrument. Refine instrument and procedures.

iv. Modify Instrument

Change concepts measured, populations studied, research application, instrumentation, or method of administration.

PRO

iii. Assess Measurement Properties

Assess score reliability, validity, and ability to detect change.
Evaluate administrative and respondent burden. Add, delete, or revise items.
Identify meaningful differences in scores. Finalize instrument formats, scoring, procedures, and training materials.

FIGURE 3-2 The patient-reported outcomes (PRO) development and modification process from Food and Drug Administration draft guidance.

Source: Reprinted from US Department of Health and Human Services FDA Center for Drug Evaluation and Research, US Department of Health and Human Services FDA Center for Biologics Evaluation and Research, US Department of Health and Human Services FDA Center for Devices and Radiological Health. Guidance for industry: patient-reported outcome measures: use in medical product development to support labeling claims: draft guidance. *Health Qual Life Outcomes.* 2006;4:79.

interviews can provide additional detailed information. Expert consensus using formal assessments such as the Delphi or nominal group methods may also be used to ensure content validity of an instrument. The details of instrument development are beyond the scope of this chapter, but interested readers can find more information in the Additional Resources at the end of the chapter. After a new instrument has been developed, the next step is to assess its measurement properties (reliability, validity, and responsiveness, discussion of which appears in the next section) and finalize its scoring algorithm and the mode of administration. Once the instrument's psychometric properties (ie, reliability, validity, and responsiveness) are established, it is ready to be used in clinical research. Because health measures derive from multiple concepts and theories, it is important to be mindful of their measurement procedures and to fully recognize their strengths and limitations.

■ Psychometric Properties

When evaluating an HRQL instrument, a main concern is the instrument's validity and reliability. Content validity is indicative of the extent to which the instrument consistently measures the constructs that it was intended to measure. Reliability is an expression of the accuracy of that measurement. The instrument must also be free of bias and distortion. Strong evidence of an instrument's psychometrics will boost stakeholders' confidence in using HRQL results in health care decision making. A key point that health care researchers should keep in mind is that an instrument's reliability and validity are specific to a particular disease/condition and population. A determination of psychometric properties falls along a continuum rather than dichotomous (eg, yes or no) indices.[22]

There is no absolute or completely valid and reliable instrument; a validated or reliable instrument implies that the instrument's psychometric properties in a target population have been assessed. A reliable instrument does not have to be valid, but a valid instrument will almost always be reliable. For example, if a scale consistently reports the same weight of 1.8 lb as 2 lb, it is reliable (consistent) but not accurate (valid). Validity, ultimately, is not a characteristic of the instrument but rather of the purpose to which the instrument is put. As a result, the same instrument may be valid in one application and not valid in another.

Reliability

Reliability is a fundamental feature that reflects the instrument's measurement error. It is the proportion of variance attributable to the true score of the latent variable as reflected in the results' reproducibility. For computing the reliability of an HRQL measurement scale in this chapter, the focus will be on item responses that are continuous or multiple-value options rather than dichotomous options (eg, yes or no) and will only consider internal consistency and test-retest reliability.

Internal Consistency

Internal consistency describes the extent to which items are homogenous in terms of relating to the same construct or domain or how well a set of items measures a single latent construct. Each domain is intended to measure a single phenomenon, and the relationship among items is logically connected. High intercorrelation in a domain suggests that the items are measuring the same thing. Internal consistency can be measured using the Cronbach coefficient alpha (α).[18] Taking depression as an example, variability among items in the same domain can have two components: true differences among depressed patients (eg, signal) and other differences caused by extraneous, non–depression-related factors (eg, noise). A reliable scale should have a high ratio of signal to noise. The proportion of total variation that is signal equals α or 1 minus the error variance, presumably the true score of a latent variable underlying the items. If the latent variable has k items, the α can be computed by

$$\alpha = \frac{k\bar{r}}{1+(k-1)\bar{r}}$$

Where $\bar{r}$ is the average inter-item correlation that represents the estimated reliability for a single item. This formula is known as the Spearman-Brown prophecy formula or the standardized Cronbach α. The possible Cronbach α value ranges from 0.0 to 1.0, where 0 represents no reliability and 1 represents perfect reliability. The degree of homogeneity, or α, should be sufficient to suggest that the items tap into the same domain, but not too high as to imply that a single item would suffice and that the instrument includes excessive respondent burden. Also, note that increasing the number of k items of an instrument (all else being equal) will, for purely arithmetic reasons, increase the reliability of the instrument.

One benefit of using a more reliable scale is the ability to achieve a greater statistical power for a given sample size, or equivalently, the possibility of using a smaller sample size to obtain a particular level of statistical power. This point is especially relevant in clinical trials, both to maximize the likelihood of discerning HRQL changes and to minimize sample size because clinical trials are time consuming and rather costly. Although there is no clear-cut number for the α, a value of 0.70 is normally a threshold for a good scale used to assess populations or groups.[23,24]

Test-Retest Reliability

The stability of an instrument can be thought of as how constant scores remain from one occasion to another (assuming that the health construct of interest remains stable). If scores show significant variance in the absence of any change in the underlying latent variable, that would be one source of noise that would reduce measurement performance. This instrument characteristic can be assessed using the *test-retest* method.[18] Typically, test-retest reliability can be done by giving items to one group of patients on two separate occasions and then determining the intraclass correlation coefficients (ICCs) between the first and second administrations. A minimum threshold criterion for a test-retest ICC would be 0.70. More stringent performance may be required depending on the application.

Although test-retest reliability is appealing because it represents instrument repeatability, factors unrelated to random errors or scale instability might cause changes in the scores when given on two separate occasions. Examples include (1) a real change in the health construct of interest, (2) a variation in the continuum of the health construct, and (3) changes in other health constructs that affect a phenomenon of interest.[25] The important point is that an ICC can meaningfully imply an instrument's reliability only if the phenomenon is constant.

Validity

Measurement validity refers to the extent to which the instrument measures what it purports to measure. Validation is a process of hypothesis testing that focuses on logic and methods to answer whether the results allow health care researchers to draw the inferences they wish to make. In this chapter, only 4 types of validity will be discussed: content validity, criterion validity, construct validity, and responsiveness and sensitivity to change.

Content Validity

Content validity concerns the evidence that a set of items in a domain indeed represents what it claims to represent. It can be determined by a systematic evaluation of whether items and response options are relevant and are comprehensive measures of the domain or construct.[4] The appropriate content that generates the items could come from patients and then be examined by a group of experts.

Criterion Validity

Criterion validity is the correlation of instrument scores with an external measure considered to be a gold standard. Criterion validity can be divided into two types: concurrent and predictive validity. Concurrent validity is a strong correlation between a new instrument and another well-accepted existing instrument when administered to a patient at the same time. Predictive validity refers to the ability of the instrument to predict future health status or disease condition. It is examined after a period of time because it requires the results from the criterion measure. However, because quite often no gold standard is available, criterion validity, while highly desirable, may not be obtainable.

Construct Validity

Construct validity includes the extent to which a measure correlates with other similar measures (convergent validity) and does not correlate with dissimilar measures (discriminant or divergent validity). It can be tested by observing (1) relationships between the items and domains if they confirm the hypotheses in the conceptual framework and

(2) results, if they distinguish one group from another based on a prespecified variable that is relevant to the concept of interest.[4] These proposed underlying factors are called hypothetical constructs because we are dealing with abstract variables, phenomena that cannot be directly observed. For example, the ability to find books on a shelf in patients with low vision can be tied to a degree of visual acuity.

These constructs are not seen directly; only their hypothesized manifestations in terms of the patients' observable behaviors are inferred. No single study explicitly proves a construct. Researchers are often able to make different assumptions based on their theory or construct. Establishing construct validity is an ongoing process in which more is constantly learned about constructs, making predictions, and testing them. Eventually, the construct of interest becomes established in a nomological network of interrelated constructs, solidifying our confidence in the construct's validity.[26]

Responsiveness and Sensitivity to Change

There is no consensus on whether responsiveness and sensitivity to change are totally separate attributes or parts of validity.[4,27,28] Whereas sensitivity to change is an instrument's ability to detect any degree of change in health status over time, responsiveness refers to its ability to measure a meaningful or clinically important change.[28] These two closely related properties are crucial when selecting an appropriate measurement instrument for clinical trials. A good instrument requires sufficient responsiveness and sensitivity to detect differences between two treatment groups or in the same group when health conditions change. The more sensitive an instrument is, the smaller the sample size required to detect a *minimally clinically important difference* (the smallest change in HRQL score that is considered meaningful or important by either a clinician or a patient).

Sensitivity to change can be measured using different indices. The most popular ones include the *Cohen effect size* (an estimation of a measure of the magnitude of change in health status; average change divided by the standard deviation of the initial measurement) and the *standardized response mean* (the ratio of the mean change in a single group to the standard deviation of the change scores). Similar to other psychometric properties, the extent to which the HRQL instrument detects changes varies by patient population and also disease severity. More details can be found in Streiner and Norman.[27] Normally, a generic HRQL instrument exhibits lower degrees of these properties when compared with a disease-specific instrument.[29] Details on generic and disease-specific HRQL instruments are further addressed in Chapter 4 to guide how to select appropriate instruments in health care research.

■ Summary

HRQL is an important feature that has grown in importance in health care decision-making processes, not only to inform physicians regarding treatment outcomes (both favorable and unfavorable) but also to assist policy makers to better allocate scarce health care resources. HRQL information obtained directly from patients is preferable in economic evaluation because patients are the primary recipients in health care. There are several reasons why HRQL assessments may be included in clinical practice and clinical trials. In clinical trials, the most obvious reason is to compare study interventions in which it is important to identify those aspects of HRQL that may be affected by the treatments. Researchers can then use HRQL assessments as screening tools to select a population of interest and also as end points in clinical trials. In clinical practice, physicians and other health care providers may use HRQL assessments to screen patients and families and then apply prophylactic interventions or treatments, as well as monitoring and evaluating tools, to maximize patients' benefits from treatments. For these reasons, HRQL information can be a crucial aid to clinical decision making.

There is no universally accepted conceptual construct for HRQL, but a consensus has emerged that HRQL is multifaceted and subjective. Therefore, a measurement instrument is required to cover different domains of health including physical, psychological, role and social, and disease-specific functioning and general health perceptions. Poorly performing instruments may lead to misleading outcomes and inappropriate conclusions, resulting in poor decisions and wasted time and resources. Still, tests of psychometric properties are only the first step in establishing the credibility of an HRQL instrument. They only tell us whether the instrument is appropriate to use in our population of interest. Repeated use and the accumulation of data showing appropriate relationships within the nomological net are what determine eventual widespread acceptance of an instrument used for a specific application.

Validity, reliability, and the ability to detect changes are crucial information that health care researchers need to know to select the best instruments in their research and practices. For clinical research, the ability of the instruments to detect change influences sample size determination. The extent to which an HRQL instrument can detect change and its reliability and validity vary by population of interest (eg, age, race/ethnicity, sex, disease/condition, severity). Which HRQL instruments to use in a clinical trial will depend on the objectives of the study and the availability of credible instruments.

■ References

1. Guyatt GH, Feeny DH, Patrick DL. Measuring health-related quality of life. *Ann Intern Med.* 1993;118:622–629.

2. World Health Organization. WHO definition of health. Preamble to the Constitution of the World Health Organization as adopted by the International Health Conference, New York, 19–22 June, 1946 signed on 22 July 1946 by the representatives of 61 States and entered into force on 7 April 1948. World Health Organization Web site. http://www.who.int/about/definition/en/print.html. Accessed June 3, 2009.

3. The WHOQOL Group. Development of the WHOQOL: rationale and current status. *Int J Mental Health.* 1994;23:24–56.

4. US Department of Health and Human Services FDA Center for Drug Evaluation and Research, US Department of Health and Human Services FDA Center for Biologics Evaluation and Research,

US Department of Health and Human Services FDA Center for Devices and Radiological Health. Guidance for industry: patient-reported outcome measures: use in medical product development to support labeling claims: draft guidance. *Health Qual Life Outcomes*. 2006;4:79.

5. Guyatt GH, Ferrans CE, Halyard MY, et al. Exploration of the value of health-related quality-of-life information from clinical research and into clinical practice. *Mayo Clin Proc*. 2007;82:1229–1239.

6. Weinstein MC, Stason WB. Foundations of cost-effectiveness analysis for health and medical practice. *N Engl J Med*. 1977;296:716–721.

7. Mehrez A, Gafni A. Health-years equivalents versus quality-adjusted life years: in pursuit of progress. *Med Decis Making*. 1993;13:287–292.

8. Nord E. An alternative to QALYs: the saved young life equivalent (SAVE). *BMJ*. 1992;305:875–877.

9. Murray CJ. Quantifying the burden of disease: the technical basis for disability-adjusted life years. *Bull World Health Organ*. 1994;72:429–445.

10. Neumann PJ, Goldie SJ, Weinstein MC. Preference-based measures in economic evaluation in health care. *Ann Rev Public Health*. 2000;21:587–611.

11. Payakachat N, Murawski MM, Summers KH. Health utility and economic analysis: theoretical and practical issues. *Expert Rev Pharmacoecon Outcomes Res*. 2009;9:289–292.

12. Brunelli A, Socci L, Refai M, Salati M, Xiumq F, Sabbatini A. Quality of life before and after major lung resection for lung cancer: a prospective follow-up analysis. *Ann Thorac Surg*. 2007;84:410–416.

13. Callahan CM, Kroenke K, Counsell SR, et al. Treatment of depression improves physical functioning in older adults. *J Am Geriatr Soc*. 2005;53:367–373.

14. Williams RA, Brody BL, Thomas RG, Kaplan RM, Brown SI. The psychosocial impact of macular degeneration. *Arch Ophthalmol*. 1998;116:514–520.

15. Soubrane G, Cruess A, Lotery A, et al. Burden and health care resource utilization in neovascular age-related macular degeneration: findings of a multicountry study. *Arch Ophthalmol*. 2007;125:1249–1254.

16. Payakachat N, Summers KH, Pleil AM, et al. Predicting EQ-5D utility scores from the 25-item National Eye Institute Vision Function Questionnaire (NEI-VFQ 25) in patients with age-related macular degeneration. *Qual Life Res*. 2009;18:801–813.

17. McIntosh L, Kymes SM, Perron BBM, Nease RF Jr, Sumner W. Truth and consequences: assessing the relationship between health and vision related quality of life. Paper presented at: The Association for Research in Vision and Ophthalmology 2008 Annual Meeting; April 27, 2008; Fort Lauderdale, FL.

18. DeVellis RF. *Scale Development: Theory and Applications*. Newbury Park, CA: Sage Publications; 1991.

19. Turner R, Quittner AL, Parasuraman BM, Kallich JD, Cleeland CS, the Mayo/FDA Patient-Reported Outcomes Consensus Meeting Group. Patient-reported outcomes: instrument development and selection issues. *Value Health*. 2007;10(suppl 2):S86–S93.

20. Mapi Research Institute. Patient-Reported Outcomes and Quality of Life Instruments Database. ProQolid Web site. http://www.proqolid org/. Accessed June 27, 2009.

21. Murawski MM. Dimension change profile analysis: a systematic approach to HRQoL instrument selection in novel applications. *Drug Inf J*. 2003;37:165–175.

22. Frost MH, Reeve BB, Liepa AM, Stauffer JW, Hays RD. What is sufficient evidence for the reliability and validity of patient-reported outcome measures? *Value Health*. 2007;10(suppl 2):S94–S105.

23. Nunnally JC, Bernstein IH. *Psychometric Theory*. 3rd ed. New York, NY: McGraw-Hill; 1994.

24. Scientific Advisory Committee of the Medical Outcomes Trust. Assessing health status and quality-of-life instruments: attributes and review criteria. *Qual Life Res*. 2002;11:193–205.

25. Kelly JR, McGrath JE. *On Time and Method*. Newbury Park, CA: Sage Publications; 1988.

26. Cronbach LJ, Meehl PE. Construct validity in psychological tests. *Psychol Bull*. 1955;52:281–302.

27. Streiner DL, Norman GR. *Health Measurement Scales: A Practical Guide to Their Development and Use*. 3rd ed. New York, NY: Oxford University Press; 2003.

28. Liang MH. Longitudinal construct validity: establishment of clinical meaning in patient evaluative instruments. *Med Care*. 2000;38(suppl 9):II84–II90.

29. Murawski MM, Miederhoff PA. On the generalizability of statistical expressions of health related quality of life instrument responsiveness: a data synthesis. *Qual Life Res*. 1998;7:11–22.

■ Additional Resources

DeVellis RF. *Scale Development: Theory and Applications*. Applied Social Research Methods Series, Vol 26. Newbury Park, CA: Sage Publications; 1991.

Fayers PM, Machin D. *Quality of Life: Assessment, Analysis and Interpretation*. New York, NY: John Wiley & Sons; 2000.

Streiner DL, Norman GR. *Health Measurement Scales: A Practical Guide to Their Development and Use*. 3rd ed. New York, NY: Oxford University Press; 2003.

US Department of Health and Human Services FDA Center for Drug Evaluation and Research, US Department of Health and Human Services FDA Center for Biologics Evaluation and Research, US Department of Health and Human Services FDA Center for Devices and Radiological Health. Guidance for industry: patient-reported outcome measures: use in medical product development to support labeling claims: draft guidance. *Health Qual Life Outcomes*. 2006;4:79.

Health Surveys (Disease-Specific and Generic Questionnaires) and Utility Assessment

Patricia van Hanswijck de Jonge, PhD
Donald E. Stull, PhD

Learning Objectives

- Differentiate between assessments of health status, symptoms, functioning, and health states.

- Understand the differences between disease-specific and generic health measures.

- Understand what makes a good quality health measure.

- Describe the differences between health status and health state preferences.

- Describe how health states are used in cost-effectiveness analyses.

- Compare condition-specific, non–preference-based measures with generic, preference-based measures for deriving health state utilities.

■ Measurement of Health and Health-Related Quality-of-Life

Indicators of health have been collected for over a century in Western countries[1] and have been a valuable part of social indicators describing the health conditions of a society. Data on births, deaths, and morbidities provide an indication of the health of a society but can only give indirect knowledge of individual health or the effect of interventions to improve individual health. Measures of symptoms, health status, and functioning, on the other hand, have been used to gain a better understanding of individual health and the efficacy of treatments for diseases. Each of these types of individual-level measures has a specific focus and lends itself to a different understanding of an individual's health, which was described in Chapter 3.

Measuring Health Status

The type of health measure that a researcher uses depends on the dimension of health that is being assessed: health status, symptoms, functional performance, health states, and health state preferences. Each of these dimensions of health is focused on different types of assessments by patients, clinicians, or both. However, the sometimes subtle differences and seemingly confusing definitions can create some uncertainty about whether and how these concepts differ. For example, health status is defined as the patient's health condition as perceived by the patient.[2] In this respect, patient-centered health status measures often explicitly measure patients' symptoms, functional performance, and health-related quality-of-life (HRQL).

Yet, although symptoms may indicate a particular health problem (eg, increased body temperature may indicate a fever, suggesting an infection), they are not in themselves indicative of health status. In this example, contextual clues may also be necessary because increased body temperature can result from physical exertion in exercise and may not indicate a poorer health status. Functional performance is defined as "the physical, psychological, social, occupational, and spiritual activities people actually *do* in the normal course of their lives to meet basic needs, fulfill usual roles, and maintain their health and well being."[3,4] There is some evidence that these dimensions of health status are not interchangeable[5] and that many of them are likely to be causally related, which can account for the correlations between them.[5,6]

Measures of health status can be (1) generic or disease specific and (2) patient reported or clinician assessed. Generic measures attempt to assess health status, overall and/or by dimension, irrespective of any disease. Disease-specific measures ask questions about health status in the context of a particular disease. Likewise, information on health status can come from patients directly or from their clinicians, who may develop their assessments from patient reports, laboratory values, and their own observations.

Patient-Reported Health Versus Clinical Assessments

The use of patient-assessed health or HRQL represents a valuable addition to clinician and clinical laboratory assessments. For some symptoms, such as pain, the patient is the only source of information about severity, frequency, and location. Clinician reports are often used as benchmarks of improvement in a patient's condition and would seem to be an acceptable approach to capturing information about patients' conditions; however, often the information clinicians have to develop their own assessments is based on information provided to them from their patients. Further, recent research indicates that the correspondence of patient- and clinician-reported outcomes of patient health is generally not high[7,8] and that patient reports of health and functioning are often better predictors of important outcomes than are clinical assessments.[9-11] Consequently, including patient-reported outcome measures in clinical trials, observational studies, or clinical practice can provide valuable insights into patients who are at risk for hospitalization, additional morbidity, or mortality.

This increased reliance on patient-reported outcomes raises issues of validity, reliability, and responsiveness of measurement as key concerns for evaluating efficacy of treatment.[12] In the areas of pharmacoeconomics and outcomes research, the development, validation, and use of patient-reported health measures have been increasingly guided by regulatory requirements, notably the US Food and Drug Administration (FDA) and the European Medicines Agency (EMA). Although these guidelines are based on long-standing psychometric practices,[13] they represent an explicit codification of practices and expectations from regulatory agencies focusing on a very narrow application of these outcomes, that is, regulatory approval of a drug or device. See Chapter 2 for the FDA drug approval process.

Generic Versus Disease-Specific Measures of Health

The choice of whether to use a generic or disease-specific measure of HRQL depends, to a large extent, on the purpose of the study. For example, generic health measures, such as the Short Form 36-Item (SF-36)[14] or the EuroQoL EQ-5D,[15,16] allow for comparison of health status and health states across many different diseases and populations. Further, some of these measures (such as the SF-36 and EQ-5D) can be used for calculating health utility scores for cost-effectiveness models (discussed later in this chapter) and for making health policy and resource allocation decisions. However, they may be less sensitive to detecting small amounts of change associated with treatment.

Disease-specific measures are designed to assess the particular symptoms, functional impairments, or consequences unique to a specific disease. Consequently, they tend to be more sensitive than generic measures to small changes in conditions associated with treatment or declines as part of disease progression. Only in some cases have disease-specific measures been used to calculate health utility values.[17] In general, these measures do not always have the qualities that allow converting disease-specific scores into preference-based (utility) scores. This is discussed in more detail later in this chapter.

Measuring Health States and Health State Preferences

Health states and health state preferences are used in cost-effectiveness studies and analyses and hence have a health economic focus. Health states, like health status, generally reflect information about multiple dimensions of health. However, in contrast to health status, health states reflect the degree or intensity across multiple domains, resulting in a unique score for each health state. Although health status measures typically have summary scores for domains or a total score, each summary score can be achieved through many combinations of scores on individual items. As with any index, two people with identical summary scores may not have identical scores on all items comprising the summary score. That is, one person can be high on one item and low on another, whereas a second person could be low on the first item and high on the second. Their summary health status scores would be identical, but this would not reflect similar health states. In contrast, and reflective of true scales, health states indicate the unique combination of scores across each domain of the measure. Thus, a health state score indicates exactly how an individual scores on each domain.

Health states reflect varying degrees of impairment or health severity, but the health state score refers to a specific combination of underlying domain scores. For example, the EuroQoL EQ-5D is one of the most commonly used generic, multiattribute, preference-based health status measures and is used to generate unique health states for each respondent (TABLE 4-1). It contains 5 domains (ie, mobility, self-care, activities, pain, and anxiety) each with 3 levels of perceived problems with each domain. Scores across all domains indicate the health state an individual reports. Thus, a health state of 11111 corresponds to the lowest level on each domain and indicates the

Table 4-1	EuroQoL EQ-5D[15,16]	
Domain		Level
Mobility		
I have no problems in walking about.		1
I have some problems in walking about.		2
I am confined to bed.		3
Self-Care		
I have no problems with self-care.		1
I have some problems washing or dressing myself.		2
I am unable to wash or dress myself.		3
Usual Activities (eg, work, study, housework, family or leisure activities)		
I have no problems with performing my usual activities.		1
I have some problems with performing my usual activities.		2
I am unable to perform my usual activities.		3
Pain/Discomfort		
I have no pain or discomfort.		1
I have moderate pain or discomfort.		2
I have extreme pain or discomfort.		3
Anxiety/Depression		
I am not anxious or depressed.		1
I am moderately anxious or depressed.		2
I am extremely anxious or depressed.		3

best health state or no problems with any domain. Likewise, a health state of 33333 corresponds to the highest level for each domain and indicates the worst health state.

Different health states representing varying degrees of impairment in these 5 domains are reflected in different health state values. A total of 243 possible health states can be defined in this way for the EQ-5D, each one uniquely identifiable. Each health state can be converted to a single value using one of the available EQ-5D value sets (United States: Shaw et al[18]; selected European Union countries: Szende et al[19]). These value sets have been derived using acceptable valuation techniques and reflect the opinion of the general population about their preference for living in each health state for a particular period of time.

Health state preferences represent the value people place on various dimensions of their HRQL or on a particular health state. Measures of health states and health state preferences are often referred to as preference-based measures, in contrast to generic or disease-specific health status measures.[20] In evaluating HRQL, it is important to make the distinction between measuring and valuing health.[21] Earlier, we discussed some aspects of measuring health. Valuing health involves establishing the relative value or importance people (eg, patients or the general public) place on different dimensions of health, different levels of each dimension of health, and different combinations of levels of dimensions (ie, health states). Health status measures, in general, are limited in their utility for economic evaluations. This is primarily because of the different goals of health status and preference-based measures. These are discussed in more detail in the next section.

■ Measurement of Health States and Health State Preferences for Use in Cost Utility Analyses

Health States, Health State Preferences, and Health Utility

A question to begin with is, "Are utilities and preferences the same?" Measurement of health state preferences and utilities has played an increasingly important role in understanding preferences individuals have for different health states or health outcomes. The terms *utility*, *preference*, *preference value*, and *preference based* are often used interchangeably in the literature. Bennett and Torrance[20] report a taxonomy to help distinguish between the concepts. *Preference* is an umbrella term for all preferences, independent of how these preferences are measured.

There are two main types of preferences, which are distinguished by how they are measured. *Values* are preferences measured under certainty; the preference measurement question does not include any risk. *Utilities* are preferences measured under uncertainty; the preference measurement question involves a risk or probability. Standard gamble is the measurement instrument that produces utilities; the preference measurement question includes an element of risk. Time trade-off and rating scales produce preference values; the preference measurement question does not include any risk.

What Are Health Utilities and How Are They Elicited?

The term *utility* in the concept of HRQL measurement refers to the desirability or preference for a health condition. There are two major methods of preference elicitation techniques: direct preference-based measures and multiattribute preference-based measures. The direct measures require the respondent to place a value on specific health states, whereas the indirect approach requires the respondent to complete a questionnaire, the responses to which are then fed into an existing utility function that assigns preference value scores based on preference scores obtained directly from the general population.

Direct Preference-Based Measures

In the direct approach to preference measurement, the respondent is asked to value a health state directly using a preference elicitation technique. There are three main direct preference elicitation techniques: the visual analog scale (VAS), time trade-off (TTO) technique, and standard gamble (SG) method.[22] Other techniques that have been used to value health states include magnitude estimation,[23] the equivalence technique (person trade-off),[24] ranking, and discrete choice experiment.[25] However, these latter techniques are applied less frequently. In this chapter, we will only be concentrating on the main methods of utility elicitation.

Visual Analog Scale   The VAS is simply a line with well-defined end points, on which subjects are asked to rate a given health state. The end points range from "full health" or "most preferred health state" to "least preferred health state" or "dead" on a 0 to 1 scale, where 0 represents states regarded as equivalent to "dead" and 1 represents states regarded as equivalent to "full health." VAS end points are required to be clear and unambiguous, with associated definition of "full health," to ensure comparability between respondents. Furthermore, the VAS requires clear calibration on the scale (ie, 0 to 10 or 0 to 100).

The respondents are asked to imagine that they would live in the designated health state, without change, for a designated time, with the same outcome at the end of all states. The respondents are asked to preference rank the states relative to each other and relative to the anchor states on the scale. The respondents may also be asked to place the states on the scale in any order, rather than being determined by "full health" and "dead" states. To encourage elicitation of interval scale values, respondents must be instructed, a priori, to place the health states on the scale so that the relative distance between the locations reflects the relative difference they perceive between the health states.

The VAS allows for valuation of health states worse than dead by asking respondents to value "dead" on the same scale along with their own health state and the various hypothetical health states of interest. Once a value has been obtained for "dead," all health state valuations are transformed using the formula:

$$A_i = R_i - R \text{ (dead)}/R \text{ (best)} - R \text{ (dead)},$$

where A_i is the adjusted VAS rating for health state h_i; R (dead) is the raw rating given to "dead"; R_i is the raw rating given to health state h_i; and R (best) is the raw rating given to "full health." The value for A_i would lie between 1.0 (full health state) and 0 (dead health state) or have a negative value for states valued worse than dead.

The Standard Gamble   The SG task is the classical approach to utility measurement derived directly from the axioms of expected utility theory (EUT) and is considered, by some health economists, as the "gold standard" for health state utility derivation.[22] EUT offers a normative framework for describing how individuals would make decisions under conditions of uncertainty if they adhere to a set of axioms.[26] Among the key axioms of EUT are the requirements that utilities are transitive and continuous. The SG is based directly on this continuity axiom and is the only method of utility derivation consistent with EUT. The SG has been widely applied in the decision-making literature, including medical decision making (valuation of health states). The SG method derives utilities for individual health states by asking patients to decide between a specific state of illness and a gamble on the alternative, complete recovery or death. The probabilities between the two alternatives are varied until a point of indifference between both alternatives is reached.

The SG task can be used to elicit health state values for states considered "better than dead" and states considered "worse than dead." For health states that are better than dead, the SG presents the respondent with two hypothetical states of health. Choice A is the uncertain choice and contains two possible health state outcomes: either the respondent is returned to normal health and lives for an additional t years (probability P), or the patient dies immediately (probability $1 - P$). Choice B is the certain choice of chronic state h_i for life (t years). The two living health states are specified as lasting a designated length of time (as in the VAS exercise) and terminating in death. The respondent is then asked to choose between the two alternatives. The probabilities of the two possible results are then varied until the subject is indifferent to both. The probability P at the indifference point can be directly interpreted as the utility of the health state choice B for the duration specified, on a scale where the utility of full health for the same duration is 1.0 and the utility of dead is 0.0 (FIGURE 4-1).

For chronic health states considered worse than dead, the SG approach is modified accordingly. Choice A is the uncertain choice and contains two possible health state

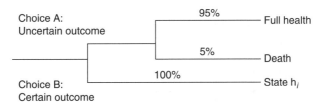

FIGURE 4-1 Example of standard gamble for states "better than dead."

outcomes: Either the respondent is returned to normal health and lives for an additional t years (probability P), or the patient remains in the chronic health state h_i for life (t years; probability $1 - P$). Choice B is the certain choice of death. In practice, the probabilities for choice A outcomes will vary toward one another until the respondent considers the odds of either outcome equally acceptable.

The Time Trade-Off   The TTO technique was developed specifically by Torrance[22] as an approximation to the SG method to overcome the difficulties that some respondents have with the notions of probabilities presented in the SG exercise. In contrast to the SG, in the TTO exercise, the respondent is asked to choose between two alternatives of certainty rather than between a certain outcome and a gamble with two possible outcomes. The SG method assesses the value of health states by asking a hypothetical question of willingness to trade that health state and its duration for the state of "full health" for a lesser number of years of life. The more debilitating the health state being valued, the more years of life a respondent would be willing to give up to attain perfect health for those years of life.

Similar to the SG task, the TTO can be used to elicit health state values for states considered "better than dead" and states considered "worse than dead." For health states that are better than dead, the TTO asks the respondent to choose between two alternatives. Alternative A is living for period t in a less than full health state (state h_i). Alternative B is full health for a period x where $x = t$. Time x is varied until the respondent is indifferent between the two alternatives. The TTO score for health state B is x/t (FIGURE 4-2).

For chronic health states considered worse than dead, the TTO exercise is modified accordingly. For health states worse than dead, the TTO asks the respondent to choose between two alternatives. Alternative A is immediate death, and alternative B is living a specified length of time (γ) in state h_i followed by x years in full health where $x + \gamma = t$. Time x is varied until the respondent is indifferent between the two alternatives. The value for state h_i is then given by $h_i = -x/(t - x)$.

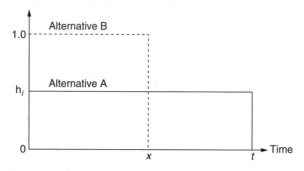

FIGURE 4-2 Example of time trade-off for states "better than dead."

In both the SG and TTO tasks, props are generally used as visual aids to enhance task comprehension, and the method of varying time/probabilities offered is designed to minimize measurement biases.[27] The specifics of the method vary depending on whether the health states being valued are chronic lifetime states or temporary states and whether the states are considered better than dead or worse than dead.

Multiattribute Preference-Based Measures

There are various generic multiattribute preference-based measures. The most widely used include the EuroQol EQ-5D,[15,16] Health Utilities Index 3 (HUI-3),[28] SF-6D,[29] Quality of Well-Being Scale (QWBS),[30,31] and Australian Quality-of-Life Scale (AQoL).[32] The EQ-5D is the most commonly used measure with agencies such as the National Institute for Health and Clinical Excellence (NICE), which recommends the use of the EQ-5D as the gold standard for preference measurement in cost-effectiveness studies, although NICE does allow the use of other relevant preference measures if justified. The HUI-3 is the second most frequently used generic preference-based measure.

Generic multiattribute preference-based measures include a system for describing health or its impact on quality of life using a standardized health classification system, as well as an algorithm for assigning values to each state described in the system. The standardized descriptive system is composed of a number of multilevel dimensions that together make up a universe of all possible health states. The algorithm is based on valuations from a sample of the general population using the SG, TTO, or VAS valuation techniques. The various generic measures differ considerably in terms of their health classification systems, the valuation methods, and the populations used to value the health states.

Whose Preferences? Patients Versus General Public

There is debate about whether preference values should be elicited from patients or members of the general public. Recently, this debate has been characterized as the choice between using health state values based on preferences versus experiences.[33,34] The choice of whether to derive preferences from patients or from the general public is important because the values resulting from these valuations have been shown to vary. Where the same health states are valued by both patients and the general public, patient values tend to exceed those derived from the general public.[35] Patients with firsthand experience of the health states being valued tend to place a higher value on dysfunctional health states than members of the general public who do not have this experience. Furthermore, the discrepancy between patient and public valuation seems to be larger when patients value their own health state.[36,37]

The variation between patient and general public valuations may be due to a number of factors. These include poor or limited descriptions of health states for the general public valuations, differences in internal standards between those who have experienced the health state and those who have not, "response shift" phenomenon, and health state adaption. Health state descriptions, or "vignettes," are limited in their ability to describe the full health state experience. Health state descriptions generally focus on a limited number of attributes, and these attributes tend to be negative aspects of the health state. As a result, respondents bring their own experiences and stereotypes to the valuation process. Given the differences between patient and general public experiences, systematic differences in health state valuation between members of the general public and patients are expected.

Another factor contributing to the variation in health state valuation between patient and general public is the "response shift" phenomenon.[38] The response shift phenomenon suggests that individuals change their own internal standards for evaluating their own health in response to changes in or increased experience with their health conditions. Response shift may be a contributing factor to systematic differences between patients and the general public in valuing the same health state.

Lastly, individuals in an ill health state tend to adapt to the health state over time (ie, they "shift"). Individuals adapt on a number of levels including psychological, emotional, and physical; their expectations lower, and their views of what matters in life change. This in turn results in patient health state valuations exceeding those of the general population. Furthermore, individuals tend to underpredict their ability to adapt to ill health,[39] so the general population valuations will focus on the initial response to developing the health state, the transition to the state, rather than what it would be like to be in that state for an extended period of time, the longer term consequences.

There are arguments for and against using either general public or patient preference values; however, ultimately the answer to this question is a normative judgment and may be predetermined by the aim of the research question. The main argument for using the general public to value health states, particularly where health care reimbursement is publicly funded (eg, Canada, United Kingdom), is based on the premise that it is the general public's resources that are being allocated in a publicly funded health care system and, therefore, it is the views of the general public that are relevant for preference value elicitation.[40] Another argument in support of using the general public versus patient values is based on the idea that the general public is not influenced by their own health state and, therefore, their decisions are not guided by self-interest. However, the disadvantage to using general public valuations is that this group of respondents generally has little firsthand experience of the health states presented for valuation and thus do not easily understand the impact of the health state on their general well-being.

The argument for using patients' values centers around the fact that patients have "lived" the health states and thus are in the best position to know the health states under valuation. Furthermore, ultimately it is the patient who will be impacted by the decisions made based on these valuations. However, using patient values may not always be practical or ethical. Some patients may be too ill or too close to death to approach, and there may be ethical concerns related to asking patients in terminal conditions to imagine scenarios involving either the risk of death or shorter life expectancies.

Ultimately, whether preference values are derived from patients or the general public will partly be driven by what the values are to be used for. It is generally accepted that if the preference values are required for resource allocation in a public system, then values should be derived from the general public. One way of bridging the gap between general public and patient valuations is to increase the amount and type of information provided to the general public in their valuation of the health state.[35,41,42]

Which Method of Utility Elicitation Is the Right Method?

Many instruments exist that can be used to elicit preference scores. Choices include whether to use a direct or multiattribute measure and which direct measure or multiattribute measure to choose. Different measures have been shown to produce different preferences in the same patient population.[43] These differences have been shown to differ systematically and significantly depending on the choice of preference-based instruments used to provide utilities.[44-47] This variability in utility estimates has an impact on cost-utility analysis (CUA) and potentially on health care decision making. It creates problems for policy makers wishing to make cross-program comparisons, given that there is no means of comparing scores generated by different measures. For this reason, some policy makers, such as NICE,[48] have introduced a reference case that has a default for a specific instrument of choice. In the following sections, we introduce the different measures and the associated considerations in choosing which one to use in eliciting preference values.

Direct or Multiattribute Preference-Based Measures

The direct preference-based measures and multiattribute methods for utility elicitation each have their own advantages and disadvantages. The generic nature of multiattribute measures allows broad comparisons among different patient groups. For this reason, NICE has indicated the generic EQ-5D as the measure of choice for eliciting health utility scores. Furthermore, the generic nature of these measures allows them to be useful in identifying unanticipated problems that may not be covered by disease-specific measures. However, their generic nature also acts as a limitation.

The multiattribute system may not capture all of the important dimensions of health for a full health state evaluation. However, the direct assessment has the advantage that it can take into account dimensions of health that may be underrepresented or omitted in multiattribute systems. For example, the EQ-5D has been shown to not be very sensitive to variations in visual acuity in age-related macular degeneration patients.[49] The disease-specific approach allows patients to define their own health state and provide a valuation of the state. Despite this being a key advantage of the direct assessment, this method of assessment is also more burdensome than multiattribute measures. Multiattribute measures impose relatively small burdens on both the respondents and investigators and thus allow for serial use.

VAS, SG, or TTO

The choice of method for eliciting direct preferences is critical because each method results in different valuations based in large part on their underlying theoretical approaches to certainty and uncertainty.[50] SG and TTO have been favored for cost per quality-adjusted life-year (QALY) analysis because of their choice-based scaling methods. This choice-based method is also recommended by NICE in its guide to the conduct of health technology appraisals.[48] Both of these techniques have factors inherent in them that influence the particular values they generate, and there is no compelling basis to select one over the other. Both TTO and SG valuation methods are cognitively difficult for many respondents, and the values elicited will reflect factors other than pure preference values. These biasing factors include attitudes to risk (SG), time preference (TTO), and aversion to loss.[51] In contrast to the SG and TTO techniques, the VAS is easy to complete and avoids some of the cognitive issues associated with the SG and TTO techniques. However, the VAS has its own biases and is subject to context effects[52,53] and end-of-scale aversion.[52-54]

Ultimately, the preference measurement technique of choice should be led by the nature of the research question and the characteristics of the disease area and health states of interest.

EQ-5D, HUI-3, SF-6D, or QWBS

As is the case when choosing between the direct measures of preference, the multiattribute measures similarly generate varying scores.[43] This variation is a direct result of the major differences in the measures' descriptive systems and associated methods of valuation. Considerations in selecting the measure of choice will include whether there is a preference for the general population valuation method, whether there is a preference for country-specific population values, and whether there is evidence of the validity of the measures in different patient groups.

Given that the QWBS is not valued using a choice-based method (VAS), it can be argued that this instrument should not be used in CUAs, which favors choice-based utility elicitation. The decision can be further narrowed by those who favor the SG or TTO valuation methodology. The EQ-5D population valuations are based on the TTO technique, whereas the SF-6D and HUI-3 valuations are based on the SG methodology (although this is indirect for the HUI-3).

Furthermore, the choice might be based on the need for country-specific population utility scores. Although all of the measures have been valued by general population samples, these surveys have not been undertaken in all countries. This is the case with NICE[55] in the United Kingdom, which requires general population values to come from their own country. A last consideration for choosing between the instruments may be the validity of the measures in the patient group of interest. However, there is little evidence on the validity of the instruments in different patient groups. Although, there is evidence to support the case that the validity of the instruments varies by patient group, it is not possible to select one measure over another in all patient groups.[21]

Converting Condition-Specific, Non–Preference-Based Measures into Preference-Based Outcomes for CUA

Often, studies do not collect information from patients using preference-based measures. Instead, when the focus initially is on demonstrating differences between groups in responsiveness, change, or severity, the researchers may use a disease-specific measure because these measures tend to be more sensitive than generic measures. Can researchers use this disease-specific information to obtain utilities? There are two main ways in which condition-specific measures can be converted into preference-based scores that can be used in cost-effectiveness models: mapping and direct valuation.

Mapping

The first possible way is to map scores from the disease-specific measure to a multiattribute utility measure. This involves the use of an algorithm that generates weighted scores, by dimension, to create an overall utility. Two possible ways that this can be done is to use an existing algorithm for comparable patients (ie, disease and severity) for the same disease-specific and preference-based measure or to conduct analyses that link (map) the relevant domain scores of the disease-specific measure to the generic preference-based measure. This second alternative, however, requires that data are collected using disease-specific and preference-based measures in the same study and the same type of patients to allow for direct mapping.

The next step is to use a regression-based analysis to link scores on the domains of the disease-specific measure with comparable domains in the preference-based measure. The regression estimates are then used as weights in other studies of similar disease and patients to generate preference-based scores. The overall process for conducting such mapping studies is beyond the scope of this chapter, and the reader is referred to other, more detailed treatments of this method.[17,56] Examples of mapping from disease-specific to generic, preference-based measures can be found in Brazier et al,[57] Kontodimopoulos et al,[58] McKenzie and van der Pol,[59] and Sauerland et al.[60]

Direct Valuation

The second method of converting disease-specific measures into preference-based scores is to conduct a direct valuation study. In the absence of an algorithm, derived from either of the approaches described earlier, researchers must use the disease-specific measure to create health states that will be valued by the general public through standard preference elicitation methods (eg, SG or TTO). In many instances, this may be the preferable approach if the domains of the disease-specific measure are not similar to those of the generic, preference-based measure. In such cases, the items of the condition-specific measure must be selected (and often reduced in number) and summarized in a way that allows development of health states that reflect the HRQL of patients with the condition of interest. In addition, item reduction is important for reducing the number of potential health states that must be valued by patients.

Methods involving classical test theory (eg, factor analysis) or item response theory (eg, Rasch analysis) can be used to reduce the number of items and provide insights into both redundancy of items and their sensitivity for measuring the condition of interest.

The next step involves creating health states based on summary information from the reduced number or subset of items. The health state descriptions are the explicit, objective statements of the patient's experience with a specific disease.[20] Because these are used as the basis of preference elicitation from key groups, particularly the general public, it is critical that the health states cover the full range of symptoms or disease experience and severity levels.

How Are Health Utilities Used?

Utilities play a central role in determining the cost effectiveness of treatments. To establish that a new treatment is as cost effective or less costly for the same outcomes requires a metric that allows direct comparison and uses preference data from the relevant group. Cost-effectiveness analysis (CEA) is a systematic method of comparing two or more alternative programs by measuring the costs and consequences of each. CUA is a specific type of CEA in which the denominator is measured in terms of QALYs gained. Utility assessment is an important part of CUA, which has been recommended for use in economic evaluations of health care interventions. CUA is similar to CEA except for its use of QALYs as the measurement of outcome in its denominator. CUA includes both the quantity of life (mortality) and the changes in the quality of life (morbidity). The quality adjustment in the QALY is based on a set of values or weights called utilities. These utilities reflect individual preferences for each health state of interest. See Chapter 13 for a further description of CUA and CEA.

QALYs are calculated by estimating the total life-years gained from a treatment and weighting each year with a quality-of-life score (from 0, representing worst health, to 1 or 100, representing best health) to reflect the quality of life in that year. The underlying concept is that an extra year of good health does not have the same value to a patient as a year in a poor health state. If a lifetime can be prolonged by a medical treatment or a patient's quality of life can be improved, this can be expressed in QALYs gained.

If the survival year is spent in perfect health, that year is multiplied by 1 and, therefore, has a full value. However, if that year is spent in a health state specified with a 0.8 utility value, that year's survival is 1×0.8, or 0.8 QALY. If, due to an intervention, all 5 years of survival have a 0.8 utility score, the total QALY for that intervention (A) is calculated as $5 \times 0.8 = 4$ QALYs. If the alternative intervention B has the same survival of 5 years but with perfect health, then the calculation is $5 \times 1 = 5$ QALYs. The incremental CUA of alternative B versus alternative A is calculated as: (Cost B − Cost A)/(QALY B − QALY A). A detailed discussion of these techniques is beyond the scope of this chapter, and the reader is referred to an excellent discussion of these methods in Brazier et al.[21]

■ Summary

Health is a complex, multidimensional construct that continues to receive much conceptual and empirical attention. These efforts are likely to continue unabated as measures of health status and health states receive increasing attention as diagnostic and prognostic indicators, and with their role as key pieces of information for decisions about treatment efficacy and cost effectiveness.

Because much of the work in health utilities has come out of the economics field, much of the development of health state preferences has not involved the same psychometric attention as measures of health status or functional health. Thus, attempts at a one-size-fits-all measure or method often result in less than optimal assessments of utility. The counterargument is that not having a uniform measure and method results in mixed comparisons and no clear standard.

At present, regulatory and reimbursement approaches in North America (especially the United States), the United Kingdom, and Europe are quite distinct. To a large extent, the use and continued refinement of the different measurement approaches described in this chapter reflect these different perspectives and goals. In countries with reimbursement systems that are largely publicly supported, evaluations of value of treatment or the lack of desirability of different health states based on input from the general public remain paramount. In private payer systems, such as the United States, these approaches have not taken hold as substantially. Instead, changes in health status, generic or disease-specific, are often used as efficacy end points in clinical trials with consideration for use in labeling claims, as opposed to reimbursement decisions.

Assessing the health status of patients, whether generic or condition-specific, and evaluating health states are directed toward different goals. Further, focusing on generic or condition-specific health status yields much different information about a person's health status. The former may allow comparisons with other conditions but may not be as sensitive to the actual experience with that disease or changes in that condition resulting from treatment. Likewise, deriving utilities from generic, preference-based measures may be less sensitive than using something more condition-specific but may not provide comparisons of value across conditions easily. Further, current preference-based measures (eg, EQ-5D, SF-6D, HUI-3) often result in very different utilities, depending on level of severity or morbidity of the condition under investigation.[28,43,61] Thus, continued work and efforts toward harmonization of these methods for assessing value for treatments is clearly needed.

As noted earlier, health and measures of health status are multidimensional. Further, there is evidence that these dimensions are causally related and not necessarily contemporaneous.[5,6] This suggests that in the context of clinical trials, it may be useful to model these lagged effects to understand more fully how diseases and their treatments affect patients and which dimensions, if any, are most salient to patients and hold the most value for the general public.

■ References

1. McDowell I, Newell C. *Measuring health: A guide to rating scales and questionnaires.* 2nd ed. New York: Oxford University Press; 1996.

2. Guyatt GH, Feeny DH, Patrick DL. Measuring health-related quality of life. *Ann Intern Med.* 1993;118:622–629.

3. Leidy NK, Knebel A. In search of parsimony: reliability and validity of the Functional Performance Inventory-Short Form. Int J Chron Obstruct Pulm Dis. 2010;5:415–423.

4. Stull DE, Leidy NK, Jones PW, Ståhl E. Measuring functional performance in patients with COPD: a discussion of patient-reported outcome measures. *Curr Med Res Opin.* 2007;23:2655–2665.

5. Stull DE, Kosloski K, Kercher K. Physical health and long-term care: a multidimensional approach. *Am Behav Sci.* 1996;39:317–335.

6. Liang J. Self-reported physical health among aged adults. *J Gerontol.* 1986;41:248–260.

7. Chassany O, Le-Jeunne P, Duracinsky M, Schwalm MS, Mathieu M. Discrepancies between patient-reported outcomes and clinician-reported outcomes in chronic venous disease, irritable bowel syndrome, and peripheral arterial occlusive disease. *Value Health.* 2006;9:39–46.

8. McColl E, Junghard O, Wiklund I, Revicki DA. Assessing symptoms in gastroesophageal reflux disease: how well do clinicians' assessments agree with those of their patients? *Am J Gastroenterol.* 2005;100:11–18.

9. Idler EL, Benyamini Y. Self-rated health and mortality: a review of twenty-seven community studies. *J Health Soc Behav.* 1997;38:21–37.

10. Spertus JA, Jones P, McDonell M, Fan V, Fihn SD. Health status predicts long-term outcome in outpatients with coronary disease. *Circulation.* 2002;106:43–49.

11. Stull DE, Clough LA, Van Dussen D. Self-report quality of life as a predictor of hospitalization for patients with LV dysfunction: a life course approach. *Res Nurs Health.* 2001;24:460–469.

12. Scientific Advisory Committee of the Medical Outcomes Trust. Assessing health status and quality of life instruments: Attributes and review criteria. *Quality of Life Research.* 2002;11:193–205.

13. Nunnally JC, Bernstein IH. *Psychometric Theory.* 3rd ed. New York: McGraw-Hill; 1994.

14. Ware JE, Sherbourne CD. The MOS, 36-Item Short Form Health Survey (SF-36): I. Conceptual framework and item selection. *Med Care.* 1992;30:473–483.

15. Brooks R, EuroQol Group. EuroQol: the current state of play. *Health Policy.* 1996;37:53–72.

16. Dolan P. Modeling valuations for EuroQol health states. *Med Care.* 1997;35:1095–1108.

17. Petrillo J, Cairns J. Converting condition-specific measures into preference-based outcomes for use in economic evaluation. *Expert Rev Pharmacoecon Outcomes Res.* 2008;8:453–461.

18. Shaw JW, Johnson JA, Coons SJ. US valuation of the EQ-5D health states: development and testing of the D1 valuation model. *Med Care.* 2005;43:203–220.

19. Szende A, Oppe M, Devlin N, eds. *EQ-5D Value Sets: Inventory, Comparative Review and User Guide.* EuroQol Group Monographs, Vol 2. New York, NY: Springer; 2007.

20. Bennett KJ, Torrance GW. Measuring health state preferences and utilities: Rating scale, time trade-off, and standard gamble techniques. In Spilker B, ed. *Quality of Life and Pharmacoeconomics in Clinical Trials.* 2nd ed. Philadelphia, PA: Lippincott-Raven; 1996:253–265.

21. Brazier J, Ratcliffe J, Salomon JA, Tsuchiya A. *Measuring and Valuing Health Benefits for Economic Evaluations.* Oxford, UK: Oxford University Press; 2007.

22. Torrance GW. Social preferences for health states: an empirical evaluation of three measurement techniques. *Socioecon Planning Sci.* 1976;10:129–136.

23. Stevens SS. Ratio partition and confusion scales In: Gulliksen H, Messick S, eds. *Psychological Scaling Theory and Applications.* New York, NY: John Wiley and Sons; 1960.

24. Nord E, Pinto JL, Richardson J, Menzel P, Ubel P. Incorporating societal concerns for fairness in numerical valuations of health programmes. *Health Econ.* 1999;8:25–39.

25. van der Pol M, Cairns J. Comparison of two methods of eliciting time preference for future health states. *Soc Sci Med.* 2008;67:883–889.

26. Von Neumann J, Morgenstern O. *Theory of Games and Economic Behaviour.* New York, NY: Oxford University Press; 1944.

27. Furlong W, Feeny D, Torrance GW, et al. *Guide to Design and Development of Health-State Utility Instrumentation.* Hamilton, Ontario, Canada: Centre for Health Economics and Policy Analysis, McMaster University; 1990.

28. Feeny DG, Furlong W, Torrance GW, et al. Multi-attribute and single-attribute utility functions for the Health Utilities Index Mark 3 System. *Med Care.* 2002;40:113–128.

29. Brazier J, Roberts J, Deverill M. The estimation of a preference-based single index measure for health from the SF-36. *J Health Econ.* 2002;21:271–292.

30. Kaplan RM, Anderson JP. The general health policy model: an integrated approach. In: Spilker B, ed. *Quality of Life and Pharmacoeconomics in Clinical Trials.* 2nd ed. Philadelphia, PA: Lippincott-Raven; 1996:309–322.

31. Kaplan RM, Anderson JP. A general health policy model: update and applications. *Health Services Res.* 1988;23:203–235.

32. Hawthorne G, Richardson J, Osborne R. The Assessment of Quality of Life (AQoL) instrument: a psychometric measure of health related quality of life. *Qual Life Res.* 1999;8:209–224.

33. Brazier J, Akehurst R, Brennan A, et al. Should patients have a greater role in valuing health states? *Appl Health Econ Health Policy.* 2005;4:201–208.

34. Dolan P, Kahneman D. *Interpretations of Utility and Their Implications for the Valuation of Health* [working paper]. Princeton, NJ: Princeton University; 2006.

35. Ubel PA, Loewenstein G, Jepson C. Whose quality of life? A commentary exploring discrepancies between health state evaluations of patients and the general public. *Qual Life Res.* 2003;12:599–607.

36. Ratcliffe J, Brazier JE, Palfreyman S, Michaels JA. A comparison of patient and population values for health states. Presentation to the Health Economics Study Group, University of Glasgow; June 2004; Glasgow, Scotland.

37. Tengs TO, Wallace A. One thousand health related quality of life estimates. *Med Care.* 2000;38:583–637.

38. Sprangers MA, Schwartz CE. The challenge of response shift for quality-of-life-based clinical oncology research. *Ann Oncol.* 1999;10:747–749.

39. Kahneman D. Evaluation by moments: past and future. In: Kahneman D, Tversky AS, eds. *Choices, Values and Frames.* New York, NY: Cambridge University Press and the Russell Sage Foundation; 2000:693–708.

40. Dolan P, Olsen JA. *Distributing Health Care: Economic and Ethical Issues.* Oxford, UK: Oxford Medical Publications; 2002.

41. Menzel P, Dolan P, Richardson J, Olsen A. The role of adaption to disability and disease in health state valuation: a preliminary normative analysis. *Soc Sci Med.* 2002;55:2149–2158.

42. Fryback DG. Whose quality of life? Or whose decision? *Qual Life Res.* 2003;12:609–610.

43. Fryback DG, Dunham NC, Palta M, et al. U.S. norms for six generic health-related quality-of-life indexes from the National Health Measurement Study. *Med Care.* 2007;45:1162–1170.

44. Marra CA, Esdaile JM, Guh D, et al. A comparison of four indirect methods of assessing utility values in rheumatoid arthritis. *Med Care.* 2004;42:1125–1131.

45. Barton GR, Bankart J, Davies AC. A comparison of the quality of life of hearing-impaired people as estimated by three utility measures. *Int J Audiol.* 2005;44:157–163.

46. Feeny D, Wu L, Eng K. Comparing short form 6D, standard gamble, and Health Utilities Index Mark 2 and Mark 3 utility scores: results from total hip arthroplasty patients. *Qual Life Res.* 2004;13:1659–1670.

47. Longworth L, Bryan S. An empirical comparison of EQ-5D and SF-6D in liver transplant patients. *Health Econ.* 2003;12:1061–1067.

48. National Institute of Health and Clinical Excellence. *Guide to the methods of technology appraisal;* 2008. www.nice.org.uk. Document number N1618, ISBN: 1-84629-741-9.

49. Espallargues M, Czosky-Murray CJ, Banback NJ, et al. The impact of age-related macular degeneration on health status utility values. *Invest Ophthalmol Vis Sci.* 2005;46:4016–4023.

50. van Osch SMC, Wakker PP, van den Hout WB, Stiggelbout AM. Correcting biases in standard gamble and time tradeoff utilities. *Med Decis Making.* 2004;24:511–517.

51. Bleichrodt H. A new explanation for the difference between time trade off utilities and standard gamble utilities. *Health Econ.* 2002;11:447–456.

52. Torrance GW, Feeny D, Furlong W. Visual analogue scales: do they have a role in the measurement of preferences for health states? *Med Decis Making.* 2001;21:329–334.

53. Streiner DL, Norman GR. *Health Measurement Scales. A Practical Guide to Their Development and Use.* 2nd ed. Oxford, UK: Oxford University Press; 1995.

54. Torrance G, Feeny D, Furlong W. Health utility estimation. *Exp Rev Pharmacoecon Outcomes Res.* 2002;2:99–108.

55. National Institute of Health and Clinical Excellence. *Guide to the Methods of Technology Appraisal.* London, UK: National Institute of Health and Clinical Excellence; 2004.

56. Brazier JE. Valuing Health States for Use in Cost-Effectiveness Analysis. *Pharmacoeconomics.* 2008;26:769–779.

57. Brazier J, Usherwood T, Harper R, Thomas K. Deriving a preference-based single index from the UK SF-36 Health Survey. *J Clin Epidemiol.* 1998;51:1115–1128.

58. Kontodimopoulos N, Aletras VH, Paliouras D, Niakas D. Mapping the cancer-specific EORTC QLQ-C30 to the preference-based EQ-5D, SF-6D, and 15D instruments. *Value Health.* 2009;12: 1151–1157.

59. McKenzie L, van der Pol M. Mapping the EORTC QLQ C-30 onto the EQ-5D instrument: the potential to estimate QALYs without generic preference data. *Value Health.* 2009;12:167–171.

60. Sauerland S, Weiner S, Dolezalova K, et al. Mapping utility scores from a disease-specific quality-of-life measure in bariatric surgery patients. *Value Health.* 2008;12:364–370.

61. Brazier J, Roberts J, Tsuchiya A, Busschbach J. A comparison of the EQ-5D and SF-6D across seven patient groups. *Health Econ.* 2004;13:873–884.

Overview of Statistical Analysis in Biomedical Research

Chenghui Li, PhD

Learning Objectives

- Discuss the statistical problems and alternative statistical approaches to estimate costs in pharmacoeconomic studies.
- Discuss the confounding and selection bias in evaluating health outcomes using observational studies and appropriate statistical methods to account for selection bias.
- Discuss different ways to present and estimate the uncertainty in the estimates.
- Discuss issues with missing data and appropriate techniques to deal with missing data.
- Discuss various statistical tests commonly used in pharmacoeconomic studies.
- Discuss some advanced statistical tools applied in pharmacoeconomic studies.

■ Introduction

The goal of this chapter is to provide an overview of statistical analysis in biomedical research. The chapter is not intended to be a review of basic biostatistics but covers some of the topics that are more important to pharmacoeconomics and health outcome research. Some advanced topics that are relevant to pharmacoeconomics and health outcome research are also discussed. For more thorough coverage of basic biostatistics, readers should refer to a good textbook on biostatistics such as those by Rosner[1] or Dawson and Trapp.[2]

■ Study Design and Bias

Study Design

Study designs in medical research can be broadly divided into three types: experimental studies, observational studies, and meta-analysis. The relative strength and weakness of each type of study design will be reviewed in more detail in Section II. In the following sections, a brief discussion of each study design is provided.

Experimental Studies

Experimental studies generally refer to randomized controlled trials. When designed and conducted appropriately, randomized controlled trials provide the strongest evidence for causality. However, randomized controlled trials are expensive to conduct because of the time and resources involved. In addition, because the focused efforts to "tease out" possible confounding factors, less representative samples may be included in the trials such that the findings may not be generalized to the patient population in clinical practice. Moreover, acknowledgment during the follow-up may introduce bias to well-designed clinical trials.

Observational Studies

Observational studies offer the opportunity to study the effects of various treatments in routine practice settings and may provide more generalizable findings compared to randomized clinical trials. They are particularly important when the intervention is known to cause harm (eg, cigarette smoking) or when treatment is withheld where known therapies are available (eg, antibiotics for an infection). In those cases, randomizing patients to interventions would be unethical. Observational studies are also important for detection of a rare event (a disease or a side effect of a new intervention) or a condition that will take a long time to develop. In these situations, randomized controlled trials often lack sufficient sample size or follow-up period to detect those events.

Observations studies are generally conducted using the following four study designs: (1) cohort studies; (2) case-control studies; (3) cross-sectional studies including surveys; and (4) case series studies or case reports. A *cohort study* starts by identifying a cohort that is free of the disease of interest and following them forward to see the development of the disease. As such, this type of study is also called an **incidence study** in epidemiology because it is designed to identify new cases from those who initially a free of the disease. Cohort studies are also **longitudinal studies** because they require subjects to be observed over time.

Cohort studies can be conducted either prospectively or retrospectively. Prospective studies collect new data after the study starts, and retrospective studies use data that have already been collected and reported previously (before the current study). When conducted prospectively, investigators have the opportunity to purposefully measure variables that may bias or confound findings, which can be controlled for later using statistical approaches. However, similar to clinical trials, prospective cohort studies can also be expensive to conduct, particularly if the disease or outcome is rare. In this case, they can take a long time to carry out and may require a large number of subjects.

In addition, attrition may lead to further bias. In those cases, retrospective cohort studies provide quicker and cheaper alternatives. Retrospective cohort studies use existing data such as administrative insurance claims databases and are less expensive to conduct since the data have already been collected prior to the study. However, since the existing databases are not collected specifically for the current study or for research purposes in general (eg, the purpose of insurance claims databases are for reimbursements), confounding and bias are more common in retrospective studies than in prospective studies and will require more extensive statistical adjustment.

Case-control studies identify patients with disease (cases) and without disease (controls) first, and then look backward to check for the exposure to a risk factor of interest in each group. As such, when a disease is rare, case-control studies guarantee that a sufficient number of patients with disease will be included in the study. However, a major challenge in case-control studies is to identify the appropriate controls. If the controls are not comparable to cases, biased results can be obtained. *Cross-sectional studies* are prevalence studies. They examine the presence of a disease or risk factor and other population characteristics at a point in time. The correlation between a certain disease and a risk factor may be explored but can only be suggestive of an association. This is because temporal order of the disease and the risk factor cannot be determined. *Case reports or case series studies* are meant to describe a new phenomenon. A case report is a report of a single patient, and case series are a collection of case reports.

Meta-Analysis

Meta-analysis is used to synthesize existing evidence. It is particularly useful when there are no large randomized controlled trials, but a number of well-designed small clinical studies have been conducted. In comparative effectiveness studies, when there are no head-to-head randomized trials, meta-analysis can be used to estimate the effects of alternative treatment options using results from placebo-controlled trials. Meta-analysis is also helpful when controversial findings exist in the literature; in those cases, meta-analysis can generate a weighted average of the treatment effect. In decision modeling analysis, meta-analysis can be used to generate values for model parameters, particularly those of effect sizes.

Validity and Bias

Obtaining valid results is always an important goal of any research. When designing medical research, it is important to ensure that the study will generate valid result. Invalid inferences or incorrect conclusions from research can occur from three sources:

- Chance
- Bias
- Confounding

Chance

Statistical inferences are based only on a sample of a population. Just by chance, one may observe a positive or negative treatment effect. The goal of statistical testing is to determine the probability that the observed treatment effect can result from chance. Random errors cannot be eliminated. However, increasing sample size will reduce error from random variation and lead to more precise estimates of the true treatment effects.

Bias

Bias results from systematic errors in the way study subjects are selected, measured, and analyzed. Unlike errors resulting from random variations, increasing sample size will not reduce the bias. Systematic errors will result in inaccurate estimates, which lead to invalid conclusions. Some design techniques such as randomization and blinding can be applied to reduce certain biases. However, no study design can prevent all biases. Therefore, it is important to recognize the limitation of the study due to potential biases. There are many types of possible biases. The following classification of the three typical types of biases is based on the stage of the research when the bias may occur.[3]

- Selection bias
- Measurement bias
- Analytical bias

Selection bias occurs when subjects selected into the sample are not representative of the population or the allocation of treatment is related to the outcome one wants to measure. There are many sources of selection bias. Sachett[4] described 35 different biases. More detailed coverage can also be found in Feinstein.[5] Dawson and Trapp[2] provided an overview of the major types of selection bias in Chapter 13. Randomized allocation of treatment may alleviate the selection bias due to treatment assignment in clinical practice. However, participants in clinical trials are self-selected and may not represent the patient population in typical clinical practices. Selection bias is particularly problematic in observational studies when the treatment assigned is not randomized and may be correlated with important prognostic variables.

Measurement bias occurs when there are systematic differences between treatment groups regarding how the outcomes are measured or reported by study participants, caregivers, or researchers. One example of such bias is when an investigator, hoping for a successful study, may unknowingly ask questions or examine patients in the treatment group in a way that may lead to a higher chance of detecting a condition of interest than the control group. This type of bias can be reduced through blinding of study participants, caregivers, and researchers. Measurement bias can also arise from inaccuracy in measurement instruments.

Bias can also occur at the end of the study when there is a difference in completion between treatment groups or crossover of assigned treatment group. Participants who changed treatment groups, who withdrew, or who were lost to follow-up may be systematically different from those who remained in the study. Biases resulting from these sources are sometimes referred to as **analytical bias**. Implementing strategies that will maximize follow-up and using *intent-to-treat analysis* by analyzing patients in the group to which they are randomized may reduce some of these biases. Analytical bias may also be introduced in data analysis or interpretations of study findings "if the investigators have strong preconceptions."[3]

Confounding

A confounding factor is associated with both the outcome and the potential risk factor but is not a consequence of the risk factor. An example of this is the association between antidepressants and mortality. This relationship is confounded by age because older people are more likely to be prescribed antidepressants but mortality risk also increases with age. However, aging is not a consequence of antidepressants use. Confounding factors, if unbalanced between treatment and comparison groups, can lead to selection bias. In well-executed randomized trials, all confounding factors are balanced across groups such that it will not result in biased estimates. However, in observational settings, without controlling for confounding factors, the true relationship between two variables may be altered and a spurious association can result even when two variables are unrelated. Known confounders such as age can be controlled easily through stratification by the confounders (if only a few of them) or multivariate statistical adjustment methods such as propensity score matching.[6,7] However, unknown confounders may still exist that will lead to biased estimates. Several approaches, such as the instrumental variable approach[8-10] and the Heckman selection model,[11,12] are available to control for selection bias resulting from latent confounders. Some drawbacks of these statistical methods are that they rely on specific assumptions that may not be applicable to the data at hand and can also be difficult to implement (eg, finding the appropriate instrument for the treatment is always a challenge).[13]

■ Probability and Uncertainty

Probabilities and Distribution

Understanding probabilities and probability distributions is essential to cost-effectiveness analysis. Not only are statistical inferences made based on probability theory, but this understanding is particularly important in decision modeling analyses for two main reasons. First, cost-effectiveness models often require modeling the long-term disease progression and transitions across different health states; during the course of disease, progressions are uncertain, which need to be modeled with probabilities. Second, inputs to cost-effectiveness measures come from either a single randomized controlled trial or synthesis of results from multiple trials or studies, measures which are based on samples of the population and therefore associated with estimation errors. To assess the overall uncertainty in the output measures (eg, incremental cost-effectiveness ratios), theoretical probability distributions are often assumed for each input in the cost-effectiveness measure, and simulations from the joint distribution of all inputs can be used to evaluate the degree of uncertainty in cost-effectiveness measures as a result of uncertainty in the source data.

I will start the discussion by providing a frequency definition of probability. Some basic properties of probabilities will be reviewed, followed by discussions of several theoretical probability distributions that are commonly used in cost-effectiveness analysis.

What Is Probability?

The frequency definition of probabilities is defined in the sense of empirical probabilities but over an indefinitely large number of trials. In other words, it is the relative frequency of an event occurring if the same trial could repeatedly be conducted over and over again. In reality, experiments cannot be performed for an infinite number of times. Instead, probability can be estimated by the sample proportions (ie, the sample relative frequency of an event from large samples).

Probabilities have several important properties:

- The probability of an event E, denoted as $P(E)$, is always between 0 and 1, that is $0 \leq P(E) \leq 1$. $P(E) = 0$ indicates event E will *not* occur with certainty, and $P(E) = 1$ indicates that event E will occur with certainty. Any $P(E)$s in between 0 and 1 indicate that the events may occur with some uncertainty.
- The total probabilities of all possible outcomes sum to 1.

Consider a simple example. Suppose a surgical treatment carries a mortality risk of 5%. If a patient receives the surgery, he may die from the surgery or survive the surgery and live. These two events cannot happen at the same time and are referred to as "mutually exclusive." Since these two outcomes include all possible outcomes of this surgical treatment, the probabilities of being alive or dead should sum to 1. Graphically, this can be seen in the diagram in FIGURE 5-1.

Conditional Probability   Now, suppose that 3% of patients who do not die from the surgery may develop complications within a week after the surgery. This is a subbranch extended out of the branch of "alive." Because the path to this point is through the branch of "alive," the probability of 3% is the "conditional probability" of complications, *conditional* on the fact that a patient survives the surgery. The notation for conditional probability of event A conditional on B is $P(A|B)$. In this case, the conditional probability of complications, or $P(\text{complication}|\text{alive})$, is 0.03.

Two important concepts in biomedical literature, sensitivity and specificity, are defined as conditional probabilities. Sensitivity and specificity are defined in the context

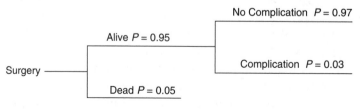

FIGURE 5-1 Mutually exclusive events.

of screening tests. **Sensitivity** is the probability of a patient with the disease screening positive for the disease. By this definition, sensitivity is a conditional probability of screening positive, *conditional* on a patient having the disease, or P(positive|with disease). **Specificity** is the probability of a healthy individual screening negative for the disease. By definition, specificity is the conditional probability of screening negative, *conditional* on a patient not having the disease, or P(negative|without disease).

Marginal Probability   If a patient came to a doctor's office for treatment advice based on the previous surgical example, what should the doctor tell the patient regarding his chance of having complications? At this time, whether the patient will survive surgery is still unknown. This probability, also called *marginal probability*, is not 3% because not all patients may survive the surgery. It is the *unconditional* probability of complication, regardless of whether the patient will die from the surgery. In general, the marginal probabilities can be derived using the following formula: $P(A) = P(A|B)$ $P(B) + P(A|\text{not } B)P(\text{not } B)$. In this example, the P(complication) = P(complication|died) P(died) + P(complication|alive)P(alive). Because it is impossible to have complications if dead, this formula is simplified to P(complication) = P(complication|alive) P(alive) = $0.03*0.95 = 0.0285$, or 2.85%. It is lower than the conditional probability (3%) because there is still the possibility at this point that the patient may not survive the surgery (ie, 5% of patients die from the surgery).

Joint Probability   Sometimes, a researcher is interested in several events occurring at the same time. This probability is called *joint probability*. If events are independent, that is, the occurrence of one event does not depend on the other, then the joint probability of the two events is simply the product of the probabilities of the two events [ie, $P(A \cap B) = P(A)*P(B)$]. This can be generalized to multiple independent events as $P(A_1 \cap A_2 \ldots \cap A_n) = P(A_1)*P(A_2)* \ldots *P(A_n)$. However, if the events are dependent, there is no general formula for the joint probabilities, which have to be derived from the joint distribution. In pharmacoeconomics and outcome research, joint probability is often encountered when conducting multivariate probability sensitivity analysis. Parameters of the cost-effectiveness model are each assumed to be drawn from a theoretical distribution and independent from each other. The uncertainty of the final cost-effectiveness measure can be evaluated through simulated samples from the joint distribution.

Probability Distributions

A probability distribution is a function that assigns probability density or mass to possible value(s) of a random variable. Probability distribution is an important concept in statistics. All hypothesis testing is based on probability distributions of the test statistics; given the probability distribution, the goal of a statistical test is to determine how likely one may observe a value or more extreme values in a sample by chance. In decision modeling analysis, probability distributions are used to assess uncertainty of the estimated cost-effectiveness measures. Each parameter is assumed to follow a certain theoretical distribution. The choice of theoretical distribution is such that the general characteristics of the distribution are consistent with that of the parameter. For instance, gamma distribution is often assumed for costs because the distribution is defined only for positive values and the distribution is skewed, both of which are typical features of cost data.

Empirical means and variances obtained from the literature or available data may be used to specify the moments of the distribution. If the estimates of the parameters are independent of each other, then the outcome can be simulated by taking random draws from each distribution. Such simulations will be carried out a large number of times (eg, 1000 times), and the frequency distribution generated from the simulations can be used to calculate the confidence intervals of the cost-effectiveness ratio. If the parameters are not independent, the dependence between parameters may be built into the variance and covariance matrix of these parameters. The confidence intervals of the cost-effectiveness measure can be calculated using the simulated frequency distribution. More detailed discussion can be found at Doubilet et al[14] and Critchfield and Willard.[15] Briggs et al[16] provide a good discussion of probability sensitivity analysis using a Bayesian approach.

Several theoretical probability distributions are often encountered in cost-effectiveness studies:

- Normal
- Binomial and Beta
- Poisson
- Gamma and log-normal

The normal distribution is the most commonly encountered probability distribution in statistics. The popularity arises not just from its mathematical properties, which make it easier to work with mathematically; more importantly, by the central limit theorem (CLT), many asymptotical distributions of sample statistics are approximately normal as the sample size gets large, regardless of the distribution in the population from which the sample is drawn. A normal distribution is symmetric, bell-shaped, and dependent on two parameters, the mean (a measure of central location) and the variance (a measure of dispersion). A variable with normal distribution can take the values of any real numbers (from $-\infty$ to ∞). The probability density function has the following form:

$$f(x) = \frac{1}{\sqrt{2\pi}\sigma} \exp\left[-\frac{(x-\mu)^2}{2\sigma^2}\right]$$

with mean μ and variance σ^2. A special kind of normal distribution is the standard normal distribution with mean of 0 and variance of 1. The probability density function simplifies to:

$$f(z) = \frac{1}{\sqrt{2\pi}} \exp\left(-\frac{z^2}{2}\right)$$

A normal distribution is often assumed for a parameter that is measured as a continuous variable unless logical constraints on the values of the parameter make it inappropriate to assume normal distribution. For instance, unit costs have to be nonnegative. In those cases, assuming normal distribution may predict values that are negative.

Beta and binomial distributions are commonly used for probability parameters. **Binomial distribution** is defined for Bernoulli trials (ie trials with two outcomes) when the trial is repeated n times and assigns a probability for any k number of successes ($k \leq n$). At an individual level, each treated patient can be regarded as an independent Bernoulli trial with an outcome of either a success or a failure and the observed data are the results of these independent Bernoulli trials; the proportion of successfully treated patients can then be used as the estimate of the corresponding probability in a model.[16] In probability sensitivity analysis, binomial distribution is often assumed for parameters that are measured as binary variables (eg, mortality). For instance, Icks et al[17] compared the cost-effectiveness of different type 2 diabetes screening strategies using a decision analytic model. In the sensitivity analysis, binomial distribution was assumed for the occurrence of glucose metabolism impairment, which was defined as a binary variable. The probability-mass function of a binomial distribution is given by:

$$\Pr(X = k) = \binom{n}{k} p^k (1-p)^{n-k}$$

where $k = 0, 1, \ldots, n$, is the number of successes out of n trials and $n - k$ gives us the number of failures. P denotes the probability of success for each trial and is assumed to be fixed. It can be shown that the mean and variance of a variable with a binomial distribution is np and $np(1 - p)$.

However, the binomial distribution is a discrete distribution related to the sample size of the study generating the data. Sometimes, it may make more sense to model the distribution of probability in the model as continuous.[16] In that case, a beta distribution is often assumed. **Beta distribution** is a continuous distribution on the interval of 0 to 1. It requires two parameters, α and β, such that the mean is $\alpha/(\alpha + \beta)$ and variance is $\alpha\beta/[(\alpha + \beta)^2(\alpha + \beta + 1)]$.[16]

Poisson distributions are often assumed for parameters that are measured as counts. Some examples of count variables are frequency of hospitalizations and visits to physicians or emergency departments. Let's denote the expected number of events per unit of time as λ. The probability of k events occurring in a time period of t for a Poisson random variable is:

$$\Pr(X = k) = e^{-u} \frac{\mu^k}{k!}$$

where $\mu = \lambda t$ is the expected number of events during time period t. A unique feature of the Poisson distribution is that the mean and variance are the same, namely, $\mu = \lambda t$.

Gamma and log-normal distributions are often used for parameters that are measured as continuous variables with known skewed distributions (eg, costs). Both are continuous distributions and are defined only for nonnegative values. A gamma distribution has two parameters, α and β, where the mean is α/β and the variance is α/β^2. Although count data can be modeled with Poisson distributions, the key assumption that mean and variance are the same may not be very applicable. One way to alleviate this problem is to further assume the mean count to have a gamma distribution. The log-normal distribution assumes that the natural log of the parameter has a normal distribution. In addition to costs, log-normal distributions are also assumed for relative risk ratios, which are often the primary outcomes in clinical trials.[16]

Uncertainty

In a cost-effectiveness study, Gold et al[18] distinguish two major sources of uncertainty: *parameter uncertainty* and *model uncertainty*. Parameter uncertainty can arise in a number of ways. First, parameters are estimated from samples of a population, which is subject to sampling variation; even if the estimates are asymptotically unbiased, the associated random errors from these estimates still lead to uncertainty in the final cost-effectiveness measure.[18]

Second, in some cases, certain key parameters may be uncertain (eg, epidemiology of disease or patterns of physician behavior and patient compliance), may not be known (eg, future inflation rate of medical care cost), may have unresolved disagreement (eg, the appropriate rate of discount for social decision), or may have no available estimates for the population of interest and need to be extrapolated from other populations, all of which will contribute to the overall parameter uncertainty.[18]

Gold et al[18] separate model uncertainty into *model structure uncertainty*, which arises when results from a cost-effectiveness study depend on the model structuring assumptions such as the relationship among parameters, and *model process uncertainty*, which can arise when different modeling process may be implemented by different analysts. The latter type of uncertainty is likely but rarely examined in practice. Gold et al[18] provide a brief discussion and some rare examples when a comparison across analysts was made. For model structure uncertainty, there is often no clear evidence which functional form best describes the relationship between parameters. In the absence of adequate data to test which assumption is more appropriate, the choice of functional form is often made based on ease of mathematical convenience.[18] Such limitation should be acknowledged in the report of the analysis. Additionally, sensitivity analysis may be conducted by computing the cost-effectiveness measure under alternative functional forms; a weighted average of the cost-effectiveness measures from computations using different assumptions may be computed with weights reflecting the degree of confidence in each structural form.[18] More detailed discussion on sensitivity analyses in decision modeling analyses can be found in Section III.

■ Estimating Risk

Relative Risk and Odds Ratio

In a cost-effectiveness analysis, effectiveness of a treatment relative to the comparison is often measured by relative risk ratio or odds ratio. To understand the difference between the two, suppose that a prospective trial is conducted to compare a new cancer treatment (n = 150) with the standard treatment (n = 200). At the end of the 5-year study period, 30 patients in the new treatment arm and 50 patients in the standard treatment arm died. For simplicity, let's assume no patients are lost during the follow-up period. This information is represented in TABLE 5-1, a 2 × 2 contingency table.

Relative risk (RR) (or risk ratio) is defined as the ratio of event rate in each treatment arm:

$$RR = \frac{\text{Event Rate [New Treatment Group]}}{\text{Event Rate [Standard Treatment Group]}}$$

In this example, the event we are interested in is death during the 5-year period after treatment.

The event rate in the new treatment arm = 30/150 = 0.20.
The event rate in the standard treatment arm = 50/200 = 0.25.

Thus, the RR is 0.20/0.25 = 0.80.

A related concept is called relative risk reduction, defined as:

$$\text{Relative Risk Reduction} = 1 - \text{Relative Risk}$$

In this example, the relative risk reduction of death is 1 − 0.80 = 0.20.

Because relative risk reduction is measured in relative terms, it may elevate the benefit of a treatment because it does not account for the level of baseline risk. To see this, let's consider a simple example. Suppose that in one study, the mortality risks are 0.05 for the standard treatment group and 0.04 for the new treatment group; and in another study, the mortality risks are 0.8 for the standard treatment group and 0.64 for the new treatment group. Both studies yield a relative risk reduction of 0.2, which makes the new treatments appear to be equally effective in reducing mortality. However, the second study generates a much larger and clinically more significant

Table 5-1	Relative Risk		
	Death		
Treatment	Yes	No	Total (Row)
New	30	120	150
Standard	50	150	200
Total (Column)	80	270	350

absolute risk reduction than the second study (0.16 vs 0.01). Thus, the absolute risk reduction should also be reported.

$$\text{Absolute} \atop \text{Risk Reduction} = {\text{Risk} \atop [\text{Standard Treatment} \atop \text{Group}]} - {\text{Risk} \atop [\text{New Treatment} \atop \text{Group}]}$$

In the previous example presented in Table 5-1, the absolute risk reduction is $0.25 - 0.20 = 0.05$. Although the new cancer treatment reduces the 5-year mortality risk by 20%, the absolute risk reduction is only 5%.

Absolute risk reduction is used to calculate the **number needed to treat (NNT)**, which is the number of patients required to prevent one adverse event such as death. NNT is calculated as:

$$NNT = \frac{1}{\text{Absolute Risk Reduction}}$$

In the example study, the NNT = 1/0.05 = 20. Thus, for every 20 patients who receive this new treatment, 1 will be saved from death within 5 years after treatment.

Odds ratio (OR) is another way to report the relative risk between two treatments. Instead of the ratio of risks between the treatment and comparison groups, the OR is the ratio of odds, as suggested by its name. The odds of an event is the defined as:

$$\text{Odds} = \frac{\text{Rate of Event}}{\text{Rate of No Event}}$$

Using the same example, the rate of death in the new treatment arm is 30/150 = 0.20 and that of survival (no death) is 120/150 = 0.8. Thus, the odds of death in the new treatment arm is 0.20/0.8 = 0.25. Note that since 150 is a common denominator in the ratio, the formula could be simplified to 30/120 = 0.25. Similarly, one can calculate the odds of death in the standard treatment arm as 50/150 = 0.33. The OR of death between the two arms is 0.25/0.33 = 0.76.

In general, if we can arrange the data as in TABLE 5-2, then:

$$RR \ (\text{Event}) = a(c + d)/[c(a + b)] \quad OR(\text{Event}) = ad/(bc)$$

Table 5-2	2 × 2 Table	
	Event	
	Yes	No
Treatment	a	b
Comparison	c	d

Choice Between RR and OR

The choice between RR and OR depends on several factors: (1) study design, (2) convenience, and (3) interpretability. RR requires the knowledge of those who are exposed to the treatment or risk factor, which is not required in the calculation of OR. For this reason, RR **should not** be used in case-control studies. Case-control studies identify subjects with a certain disease or outcome first; for comparison purposes, select control groups "match" closely to the disease group and therefore will not include all of those without the disease or outcome. The exposure to a certain treatment or risk factor within each group will be examined retrospectively. As such, the total number of individuals who are exposed could not be determined from such a study design. In case-control studies, the OR of having an exposure can be calculated between a disease and a control group, and the association of disease and risk factor can be tested using OR. Another reason that OR may be chosen over RR is that many studies conduct multivariate analysis to control for multiple confounders and/or reduce variation in the estimates. A common multivariate analysis tool is the logistic regression model, which reports ORs. On the other hand, RR is more often reported in randomized controlled trials without multivariate analysis because it is more intuitive and easier to interpret.

Inferences Using RR or OR

Both RR and OR are measured as ratios. A ratio of 1 means the numerator and denominator are equal. For RRs and ORs, this means that the event rates or odds of events are equal for the treatment and control groups and, therefore, there is no difference in effectiveness. Thus, to test the hypothesis of a treatment effect, the null hypotheses for both RR and OR are against 1. If RR or OR is significantly different from 1, then it indicates a treatment effect. An RR or OR that is greater than 1 indicates a higher risk, and a value less than 1 indicates a lower risk, compared to the standard treatment or placebo.

However, whether there is a real treatment effect needs to be determined through statistical tests. Statistical significance of RRs or ORs can be determined using either the P values or confidence intervals (CIs) of RRs and ORs. A P value is the probability of observing the value of the sample statistic (in this case, the RR or OR) or a more extreme value by chance. If the P value is less than the prespecified significance level (eg, $\alpha = 0.05$), then it indicates the observed treatment effect is statistically significant. The same inferences could be made using CIs of RRs or ORs. $a\%$ CIs are the range of values within which the true RR or OR lies $a\%$ of the times if we repeatedly draw samples of the same size as our study sample and recalculate RR or OR for each sample. The $a\%$ is equivalent to a significance level of $(1 - a)$. For instance, hypothesis testing using 95% CI is equivalent to a two-sided test using $P < 0.05$. To test the statistical significance, one will check to see if the CI of RR or OR includes 1. If it includes 1, then the treatment effect is not statistically significant. If the interval does not include 1, that is, either the lower bound of the CI is greater than 1 (significant positive treatment effect) or the higher bound of the CI is less than 1 (significantly negative treatment effect), the treatment effect is statistically significant.

Incomplete Data

In many randomized controlled trials or prospective observational studies, patients are followed for an extended period to compare the development of a clinical or medical event (such as death, a diagnosis of certain disease, or hospitalization). It is fairly common to have subjects lost to follow-up before the end of the study period. Attrition may arise from situations that are not likely to bias the outcome. For example, patients may relocate to another geographic location such that follow-up is impossible or may die from causes not of interest to the study (eg, accident). More often, attribution arises when subjects either experience adverse effects from the treatment or a lack of treatment effect. In these situations, ignoring those subjects or using complete case analysis will bias the results. To maintain the balance created by randomization, RR should be calculated using the *intent-to-treat* principle by analyzing all subjects in the group to which they were randomized.

Logistic Regression and Adjusted OR

In most observational studies, the relationship between a risk factor and an outcome is confounded and statistical adjustment is needed to obtain unbiased estimates. Statistical adjustment is also used to estimate the effect of other factors that may affect the outcome even if they do not confound the relationship between the risk factor of interest and the outcome. In those cases, adjustment of these factors reduces variations in the estimates. Statistical adjustments could also be made in randomized controlled trials when randomization fails to balance baseline characteristics across comparison groups or to increase precision even when randomization was successful. To adjust for multiple risk factors or confounders, regression analysis is often used.

Regression analysis is used to examine the association of multiple factors [independent variables including an indicator(s) for the treatment group(s)] with an outcome variable (dependent variable). A regression model estimates the association between a treatment/risk factor and an outcome variable, *after adjusting for all of the other confounders or risk factors* that are measured. If the outcome of interest is measured as a dichotomous variable (eg, mortality), the most commonly used regression analysis is *logistic regression*. Treatment effects in a multivariate logistic regression analysis are reported as adjusted ORs. Adjusted ORs are often different from the unadjusted ORs because of the effects of confounders.

For example, Harris and Wynder[19] conducted a study to examine the association between alcohol consumption and breast cancer in women. Without adjusting for confounders, alcohol consumption is associated with statistically significant ($P < 0.10$) increases in risk of breast cancer for all 3 levels of alcohol consumptions compared with no consumption in the group with a body mass index (BMI) of less than 22 (Table 3 of the article). However, after adjusting for confounders such as age, year of interview, education, employment, marital status, and smoking status, the associations are no longer statistically significant, and the magnitude of ORs is reduced. This suggests that the difference in breast cancer risk between the alcohol users and nonusers in this

BMI group can be attributed largely to the differences in the confounders between users and nonusers rather than alcohol consumption itself.

Survival Analysis

Let's consider the following scenario. A randomized controlled trial was conducted to compare the effectiveness of 2 new cancer treatments. Ten patients were randomly assigned to each treatment (ie, 10 to treatment 1 and 10 to treatment 2) and followed for 5 years. Five patients in the treatment 1 group died within a year and the rest survived until the end of the 5-year period. No deaths occurred in the treatment 2 group until the last year, when 5 patients died. Which drug is more effective? If one calculates the RR using the formula in the previous section, the two treatments will appear equally effective; but clearly, the second treatment is more beneficial in prolonging life. This simple example demonstrates that not only does it matter *whether* an event occurs, but also *when* it occurs, or the time to event, matters. This is particularly important for diseases such as some cancers for which there is no cure, but delaying recurrence and prolonging life are important.

Survival analysis is specifically designed to study time to an event. It can also be used to examine prognosis of disease. Additionally, it allows for comparisons among cohorts and can examine multiple risk factors or adjust for multiple confounders. Although the name suggests mortality as the outcome, survival analysis can be used to analyze a variety of clinical and medical events besides mortality. In these situations, survival simply means absence of any events of interest since the start of the study period.

In the following section, I will give a brief introduction of the basic concepts and provide a nontechnical summary of the two most commonly used techniques in survival analysis: the Kaplan-Meier method and Cox proportional hazards regression analysis.

Censoring

Censoring is used to describe the phenomenon that the time to an event is not completely observed. Because patients are followed for an extended period to compare the development of a clinical or medical event, censoring is very common. FIGURE 5-2 illustrates different ways of censoring in a clinical study. An "X" in the figure indicates that an event has occurred.

The first patient experienced the event during the study period. His/her time from the start of the study to the occurrence of the event was completely observed. Therefore, the time to the event for this patient was not censored. The second patient stayed in the study during the entire study period. Although we observed this patient from the start to the end of the study, the patient never experienced an event. After the study ended, the patient was no longer followed and we don't know whether and when the patient experienced an event. Therefore, this patient's time to event was censored. The last two patients did not complete the study and were lost before they experienced an event. Therefore, their times to event were also censored. All three phenomena describe

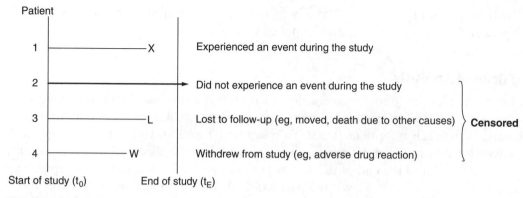

FIGURE 5-2 Censoring.

right censoring. In randomized controlled trials, only right censoring is possible because the start of exposure is observed. However, in some observational studies, *left censoring* may occur when the initial exposure to a risk factor is unknown. If both the start and end times are not observed, the time to event is referred to as a *truncation*. Both *left censoring* and *truncation* are less common and more complicated to deal with. Discussion of techniques for dealing with these types of censoring is beyond the scope of this chapter. Jacqmin-Gadda et al[20] provides a discussion of left censoring with an application to viral load in human immunodeficiency virus infection. A more comprehensive coverage of censored and truncated data in survival analysis can be found in Klein and Moeschberger.[21]

Survival Function and Hazard Rate

Survival function and hazard rate are related concepts in survival analysis. They are equivalent ways of describing the risk of a person experiencing an event over time. Survival function gives us the probability that one will survive beyond time t, which is usually measured from the start of the study period and, depending on the progression of the disease, can be measured in various increments such as weeks, months, or years.[22]

Hazard rate is the instantaneous risk of having an event at any given time t, conditional on a person having "survived," or not experienced an event prior to or at time t. It is regarded as a *rate* rather than a *probability* because it can be greater than 1.[23] Allison[23] suggests two ways to interpret hazard rates. For repeatable events, such as fractures or falls, the hazard rate can be interpreted as the number of events per person per interval of time. For non-repeatable events like death, such interpretation does not apply. Instead, Allison[23] suggested to interpret the reciprocal of the hazard rate as the expected length of time until an event occurs, assuming the hazard rate will stay the same over the interval of time. For instance, if the hazard rate for death is 0.1 per year for a 60-year-old man with diabetes and heart disease, then we can expect him to live for another 10 years assuming the hazard rate remain unchanged over the next 10 years. This interpretation is also useful for repeatable events. Both interpretations, however, provide us intuitively with the meaning of the estimated hazard rates. In reality, the hazard rate may vary over time. Our expectation of the survival will have to be adjusted accordingly over time.

Survival Analysis Techniques

Kaplan-Meier method and Cox proportional hazards regression model are the two most widely used techniques for performing survival analysis.

Kaplan-Meier Method   The Kaplan-Meier (KM) method is used to estimate the survival function. At each observational period, the KM method estimates the *cumulative survival probability* as the product of all the conditional probabilities of surviving each observed period.[22] The mathematical form of the cumulative survival function denoted as $S(t)$ is given by the following expression:

$$S(t) = P_1 * P_2 * ... * P_t$$

P_i is estimated as the proportion of subjects who did not experience an event at time i, conditional on that the subjects have not experienced the event or been censored prior to that time.

The KM estimates of the survival probabilities are often presented as KM curves, which plot the estimated cumulative survival probability or its complement (ie, 1 − cumulative survival probability) as a step function of time for each treatment group. The difference in estimated survival function across different treatment groups can be tested using log-rank tests. Log-rank tests, which are large-sample χ^2 tests, are used to compare the overall survival across treatment groups under consideration.[24] If the resulting P values for the log-rank tests are less than the specified significance level, usually 0.05, then this indicates statistically significant differences in overall survival across comparison groups. There are several variations of log-rank tests (eg, Wilcoxon, Tarone-Ware, Peto, and Flemington-Harrington tests), which differ in the weights applied to observations at different time points and may be more applicable than log-rank tests when more or less incidences occur during earlier or later parts of the study.[24]

Cox Proportional Hazards Regression Model   Although the KM method can provide an estimate of the survival function, it does not take into account various patient characteristics that may affect the risk of experiencing an event over time. For instance, is there a difference in risk of mortality between males and females? How would the treatment effect of a new drug be different between normal and overweight patients? To assess the effect of characteristics or "tease out" the confounding effect of factors to get a "true" treatment effect, the Cox proportional hazards model can be used.

As reflected in its name, a key assumption of Cox proportional hazards models is that of *proportional* hazards. The basic Cox model assumes that the hazard function has the following form:

$$h(t) = h_0(t)\exp(\beta * X)$$

Essentially, this equation states that the hazard function can be separated into two parts: a baseline hazard, $h_0(t)$, which depends only on time; and $\exp(\beta * X)$, which is a function of a set of explanatory variables X, such as patient demographic and clinical characteristics, which are assumed to be invariant over time. Now, suppose we only include one explanatory variable in X, an indicator for patients' sex: $X = 1$ if male and $X = 0$ if female. The hazard ratio between male and female patients is:

$$\frac{h(t \mid X = 1)}{h(t \mid X = 0)} = \frac{h_0(t)\exp(\beta * 1)}{h_0(t)\exp(\beta * 0)} = \exp(\beta)$$

It can be seen from this equation that the hazards are proportional and independent of time, t. Because the baseline hazards cancel out from the ratio, the Cox proportional hazards model makes no specific assumptions about the functional form of the baseline hazard other than that it cannot be negative and estimates the model by maximizing a partial likelihood function. Because of this assumption, Cox proportional hazards models are often regarded as *semiparametric* models.

Before applying a Cox proportional hazards regression model, the assumption of proportional hazards should be tested. A direct test is a log-log plot, which plots the log of the survival function against each key covariate; if the logs of the survival functions are approximately parallel across different categories of the key covariate, it is a good indication that the assumption holds. An indirect way of testing is to include the product of a covariate and time t as an additional covariate and rerun the regression model. As obvious from the expression of the hazard function, the covariates are necessarily assumed to be independent of time in order to maintain the proportional hazards assumption. Thus, a significant coefficient of the product term is an indication that the proportional hazards assumption may not hold. In such cases, the Cox model should be extended to include time-variant (or time-dependent) variables.[23,24]

The Cox proportional hazards models are mostly used to examine the time to the first event, but can be extended to model repeated events (eg, exacerbations of patients with chronic obstructive pulmonary disease) and competing risks (eg, a patient may die from a stroke or cancer, but only one actually occurs). Discussions of these extensions are beyond the scope of this chapter. Readers are recommended to consult Allison[23] and Kleinbaum and Klein[24] for a practical introduction of these models using statistical analysis software such SAS, SPSS, and STATA.

■ Estimating Mean Cost

An important component of cost-effectiveness analysis is the difference in cost for the treatments under comparison. Depending on the perspective taken by the analysis, resources used in cost calculation may differ. For example, if the analysis is conducted from a payer's perspective, then only resources covered by the payer would be included. However, if a broader societal perspective is taken, then all costs should be considered, including cost of lost time from work by patients and caregivers if both worked. For a detailed discussion of various costs that should be considered in studies with different perspectives, readers are referred to Gold et al[18] and Drummond et al.[25]

Economic evaluations are generally performed using two approaches.[26] One approach is through decision analysis modeling using data on efficacy and safety from randomized controlled trials and costs from secondary, nonclinical sources.[26] Another approach that is gaining popularity is to use health care utilization data collected on individual patients prospectively as part of a randomized controlled trial.[27] The health care utilization data are then multiplied by the appropriate unit price obtained from various secondary databases to generate a measure of the total cost for each patient.[26,28] In the second approach, more conventional methods of statistical inference are used to quantify the uncertainty due to sampling and measurement error.[26] The discussion in this section focuses on the statistical issues associated with the second approach. Nonetheless, these issues are also relevant in the modeling approach when the unit cost has to be estimated to populate the model and some primary data are available to the analyst either from an appropriately conducted randomized controlled trial or observational study to estimate the unit cost. For quantifying uncertainty in modeling approach, readers are referred to Briggs et al,[29] Gold et al,[18] and O'Brien[30] for more detailed discussion.

Two distinct features of health care costs complicate statistical inferences. One is the *skewness* in the distribution of costs data resulting from the unequal distribution of health care resources, with a small proportion of "sicker" patients using significantly more health care services than the majority of patients who may use little or no health care services. Another feature of the costs data is the *excessive zeros* resulting from a sizable proportion of individuals who may be healthy and use no health care services during a given year. This is particularly problematic when examining services such as emergency room visits or inpatient care, where as much as 80% of the population may have no visits during a year. The following discussion will review some of the commonly used statistical methods to account for these two features in the costs data.

Estimating Mean Cost and Statistical Tests: Mean Cost or Median Cost?

When the distribution is significantly skewed, a general recommendation is to use the median instead of arithmetic mean because the latter may not be a good representation of the central tendency. This is because a few extremely large or small values can significantly increase or decrease the value of the mean but will have little effect on the median. However, in economic analysis, it is recommended that mean costs should be estimated instead of median.[31] This is because decision making requires estimates of the total costs, which can be obtained by the product of mean cost and quantity of health care services used.[26] Median costs will not give us the total costs. For the same reason, the hypothesis testing based on descriptive statistics other than mean is not desirable because a significant difference in median or ranks of data may not translate into a significant difference in mean costs.[31]

Transformation and Smearing

In the presence of high levels of skewness, a common practice is to perform data transformation such that the transformed data may be less skewed and approximately normal. Several transformations are commonly used: logarithm, Box-Cox, and square root. However, these transformations provide estimates on a scale that is not relevant to a decision maker.[26] For instance, what does it mean if one found that the new treatment significantly increases the log of health care costs by 1.5 units? Reverse transformation back to the original units is needed for meaningful interpretation. However, direct reverse transformation will produced biased estimates because the mean of the reverse-transformed data will generally differ from the mean of the raw data. Duan[32] provides a smearing factor for log-transformed data when the error terms in the regression are homoscedastic. The smearing factor, which is the average of the exponential of the error terms from the regression analysis using transformed data, is then applied to the mean of predicted reverse-transformed data to correct for the bias.[32] This correction becomes cumbersome and, in some cases, impossible when the error terms are heteroscedastic in continuous or multiple covariates. For more detailed discussions, see Manning,[33] Mullahy,[34] Manning and Mullahy,[35] and Thompson and Barber.[36]

Generalized Linear Model

A recommended alternative approach is to use the generalized linear model (GLM) approach.[31] Instead of applying transformation to the cost data and conducting data analysis of the transformed data, GLM performs transformation of the mean cost directly. This way, the reverse transformation will generate no bias in the estimated mean cost. GLM also permits inclusion of covariates such as demographic characteristics and comorbidities to affect the mean costs. Although randomized controlled trials, if conducted correctly, will generate well-balanced treatment arms in their baseline characteristics, multivariate analysis may still be beneficial to reduce variation in the estimate.

The GLMs can be estimated using statistical software. For instance, researchers can fit a GLM model using either PROC GENMOD in SAS or GLM command in STATA. Estimation of a GLM generally requires an analyst to specify two things: the *link function*, which is the transformation that will be performed on the mean cost, and the *distribution function*, which is the distribution function of the random errors

Table 5-3	Distribution Functions and Commonly Used Link Functions in GLM	
Model	Link Function	Distribution Function
Linear	Identity	Normal
Logistic	Logit	Binomial
Poisson	Log	Poisson
Gamma	Log	Gamma

in cost data. Many commonly used regression models can be expressed as a GLM model with proper combinations of link functions and distribution functions. TABLE 5-3 includes the specific link functions and distribution functions for several commonly used regression models.

Linear regression is a special case of a GLM with a link function of an identify function (ie, no transformation is needed because it is already linear) and normal distribution for random error terms. For costs, gamma distribution and log link function are often chosen because gamma distribution is defined only for positive values and the distributions are generally skewed, both of which fit the typical characteristics of cost data. Manning and Mullahy[35] and Basu et al[37] compared several alternatives for estimating costs: ordinary least squares on the natural log-transformed data, GLM variants, and the Cox proportional hazards model. Although no single model is best under all circumstances, the authors found the gamma regression model with a log link more robust to alternative data-generating mechanisms.[37]

Two-Part Model

As discussed earlier, another feature of the cost data is excessive zeros. A common approach to account for excessive zeros is the two-part model.[38] As the name suggests, the analysis is conducted in two parts. In the first part, a probit or logit model will be estimated to determine the probability of having zero costs, p. In the second part, only individuals who have incurred some health care costs will be used in the analysis. Their health care costs can be estimated using GLM to account for the skewness in the data. From the second part, the mean cost is estimated and is denoted as c_u to indicate that it is based on cost among users of health care services only. The mean cost among all individuals, users and nonusers combined, can be estimated as a weighted mean of average costs in each group:

$$p^* c_n + (1-p)^* c_u$$

where c_n denotes the average health care costs among nonusers. Because nonusers did not use any health care services, c_n is 0. Thus the formula is simplified to $(1-p)^* c_u$. More discussions of the two-part models can be found in Mullahy[34] and Deb and Trivedi.[38]

Censored Cost Data

In clinical trials, it is fairly common for participants to be lost to follow-up before the end of the study period. Patients may also die during the study period if the trial is studying diseases or conditions that may be associated with high mortality. Unlike the data on time to events, censoring and costs often cannot be assumed to be independent.[39] For example, those with a lower hazard rate also accumulate costs slower. Many studies do not account for censored cost data appropriately.[31] In the following, I will review two methods that have been proposed to account for censoring on costs: the direct method proposed by Lin et al[39] and the inverse-probability weighting method.[40-44] O'Hagan and Stevens[45] compare the estimators developed by Lin et al[39] and Bang and Tsiatis[40] and provide some general recommendations on the appropriate estimation of mean costs in the presence of censoring. When adjustment for covariates in cost is needed, analysts may consider methods developed by Lin[41,42] and Jain and Strawderman.[46]

Direct Method

The direct method was first proposed by Lin et al.[39] Under certain conditions, the estimators are consistent and asymptotically normal. Lin et al[39] proposed two forms of estimators depending on how detailed the cost data are. If costs are only available when the patient experiences an event, when the patient is censored, or at the end of the study period, whichever comes first, then the data are referred to as *minimal cost data*; if costs are measured at fixed intervals (eg, weekly, monthly, annually), then they are considered as *interval cost data*.[45] For interval cost data, the method requires dividing of the duration of interest into k intervals according to these fixed observation points. The average incremental costs measured as the difference in costs between one observation point and the previous one will be calculated among those who are still at risk (ie, those who have not experienced an event and who were not censored prior to that observation point). The average incremental cost of each interval will be weighted by the probabilities for surviving up to the beginning of that time interval estimated using the KM estimator, which was discussed earlier. Overall costs are estimated as a weighted sum of the average costs in each time interval. This method assumes that subjects will contribute to the calculation of costs up to the point when they either experience an event or are censored. If only minimal cost data are available, this is reduced to the weighted average costs among those who are not censored. Since data of the censored observations are not used in the calculation of minimal cost data, this latter estimator is not efficient.[45] The estimator provided by the direct method is consistent only if the censoring occurs at the boundaries of the intervals.[26]

Inverse-Probability Weighting

An alternative method for estimating mean cost in the presence of censoring is the inverse-probability weighting (IPW) approach. Similar to the direct method, the study period of interest is also partitioned into k intervals. The IPW method uses the inverse of the probability of *not* being censored to weight the observed cost data among those who are not censored at each interval. The rational is that, if censoring is at random, then the mean cost of those who are censored can be estimated using those who are not censored. Thus, the proportion (denoted as *s*) of subjects who are not censored at interval *k* represent 1/*s* individuals during that interval. Inflating the observed costs by 1/*s* therefore will account for those who are censored at interval *k*, if censoring is at random. The probability of not being censored can be estimated by the KM estimator. Unlike the estimator provided by the direct method, the IPW estimator is consistent, regardless of the pattern of censoring.[26] More discussions can be found in Baser et al,[47] Willan and Briggs,[26] and Curtis et al.[48]

Uncertainty

Often, unit costs estimated from multiple sources are used to multiply utilization data obtained in clinical trials for each individual; with this approach, the standard errors and CIs of the mean cost are inaccurate because it does not account for the variations in estimating the unit costs from other sources. In addition, the often significant skewness in the costs data may jeopardize the assumption of normality on which the conventional CIs are based.[31] Nonparametric bootstrap methods are increasingly recommended for reporting the uncertainty and for statistical testing in mean costs.[31] The bootstrap method randomly selects samples of the same size with replacement from the study sample and reestimates the mean cost from each sample. This sampling process is repeated a large number of times. The empirical distribution of the mean costs from the samples is used to construct the 95% CIs, which are the intervals that include the central 95% of the mean costs in the constructed distribution of mean costs. For stable estimates of CIs, Willan and Briggs[26] recommend between 2000 to 5000 resamples. For more complete discussion of the bootstrap method, see Efron and Ribshirani.[49]

■ Summary

In this chapter, I provided a brief review of statistical analysis in biomedical research with the emphasis on statistical issues relevant to pharmacoeconomics and health outcome research. The discussion started with an overview of the basic study design and source for errors in measurement that could threaten the validity of study findings. It followed by a review of basic properties of probabilities and various theoretical probability distributions commonly encountered in pharmacoeconomics and health outcome research. Next, I reviewed the basic measure of risk and the regression analyses to adjust for differences in baseline characteristics across comparison groups. Finally, issues associated with estimating costs when conducting economic analyses alongside a clinical trial were also reviewed. This chapter was not intended to provide an overview of basic biostatistics. For more thorough coverage of basic biostatistics, readers should refer to a good textbook on biostatistics such as those by Rosner[1] or Dawson and Trapp.[2]

■ References

1. Rosner B. *Fundamental Biostatistics*. 6th ed. Belmont, CA: Thomson Higher Education; 2006.
2. Dawson B, Trapp R. *Basic & Clinical Biostatistics*. 4th ed. New York, NY: McGraw-Hill Companies; 2004.

3. Yamamoto ME. 2008. *Analytic nutrition epidemiology.* In Monsen ER and Horn LV (eds), Research: Successful Approaches (3rd ed), 81–89. American Diabetic Association.

4. Sachett DL. Bias in analytic research. *J Chron Dis.* 1979;32:51–63.

5. Feinstein AR. *Clinical Epidemiology: The Architecture of Research.* Philadelphia, PA: WB Saunders; 1985.

6. Rosenbaum PR, Rubin DB. The central role of the propensity score in observational studies for causal effects. *Biometrika.* 1983;70:41–55.

7. Cochran W, Rubin DB. Controlling bias in observational studies: a review. *Sankyha.* 1973;35:417–446.

8. Angrist JD, Krueger AB. Instrumental variables and the search for identification: from supply and demand to natural experiments. *J Econ Perspect.* 2001;15:69–85.

9. Angrist JD, Imbens GW, Rubin DR. Identification of causal effects using instrumental variables. *J Am Stat Assoc.* 1996;81:444–455.

10. Newhouse J, McClellan M. Econometrics in outcomes research: the use of instrumental variables. *Ann Rev Pub Health.* 1998;19:17–34.

11. Heckman JJ. The common structure of statistical models of truncation, sample selection, and limited dependent variables and simple estimator for such models. *Ann Econ Social Measure.* 1976;5:475–492.

12. Heckman JJ. Sample selection bias as a specification error. *Econometrica.* 1979;47:153–161.

13. Staiger D, Stock J. Instrumental variables regression with weak instruments. *Econometrica.* 1997;65:557–586.

14. Doubilet P, Begg CB, Weinstein MC, et al. Probabilistic sensitivity analysis using Monte Carlo simulation. A practical approach. *Med Decis Making.* 1985;5:157–177.

15. Critchfield GC, Willard KE. Probabilistic analysis of decision trees using Monte Carlo simulation. *Med Decis Making.* 1986;6:85–92.

16. Briggs AH, Goeree R, Blackhouse G, O'Brien BJ. Probabilistic analysis of cost-effectiveness models: choosing between treatment strategies for gastroesophageal reflux disease. *Med Decis Making.* 2002; 22:290–308.

17. Icks A, Haastert B, Gandjour A, et al. Cost-effectiveness analysis of different screening procedures for type 2 diabetes: The KORA Survey 2000. *Diabetes Care.* 2004; 27(9): 2120–2128.

18. Gold MR, Siegel JE, Russell LB, Weinstein MC, eds. *Cost-Effectiveness in Health and Medicine.* New York, NY: Oxford University Press; 1996.

19. Harris RE, Wynder EL. Breast cancer and alcohol consumption: a study in weak associations. *JAMA.* 1988;259:2867–2871.

20. Jacqmin-Gadda H, Thiebaut R, Ghene G, Commnges D. Analysis of left-censored longitudinal data with application to viral road in HIV infection. *Biostatistics.* 2000;1:355–368.

21. Klein JP, Moeschberger ML. *Survival Analysis: Techniques for Censored and Truncated Data.* New York, NY: Springer-Verlag Telos; 1997.

22. Linden A, Adams JL, Roberts N. Evaluating disease management program effectiveness: an introduction to survival analysis. *Dis Manag.* 2004;7:180–190.

23. Allison PD. *Survival Analysis Using SAS: A Practical Guide.* Cary, NC: SAS Institute; 1995.

24. Kleinbaum DG, Klein M. *Survival Analysis: A Self-Learning Text.* 2nd ed. New York, NY: Springer Science and Business Media; 2005.

25. Drummond MF, O'Brien BJ, Stoddart GL, Torrance GW. *Methods for the Economic Evaluation of Health Care Programmers.* 2nd ed. Oxford, UK: Oxford University Press; 1997.

26. Willan AR, Briggs AH. *Statistical Analysis of Cost-Effectiveness Data.* West Sussex, England: John Wiley & Sons Ltd; 2006.

27. Mahadevia PJ, Strell J, Kunaprayoon D, Gelfand E. Cost savings from intravenous immunoglobulin manufactured from chromatography/caprylate (IGIV-C) in persons with primary humoral immunodeficiency disorder. *Value Health.* 2005;8:488–494.

28. Barber JA and Thompson SD. Analysis and interpretation of cost data in randomized controlled trials: review of published studies. *BMJ* 1998;317: 1195–1200.

29. Briggs AH, Sculpher MJ, Buxton MJ. Uncertainty in the economic evaluation of health care technologies: the role of sensitivity analysis. *Health Econ.* 1994;3:95–104.

30. O'Brien BJ. Economic evaluation of pharmaceuticals: Frankenstein's monster of vampire of trials? *Med Care.* 1996;34:DS99–DS108.

31. Doshi JA, Glick HA, Polsky D. Analysis of cost data in economic evaluation conducted alongside randomized controlled trials. *Value Health.* 2006;9:334–340.

32. Duan N. Smearing estimate: a nonparametric retransformation method. *J Am Stat Assoc.* 1983;78: 605–610.

33. Manning WG. The logged dependent variable, heteroscedasticity, and the etransformation problem. *J Health Econ.* 1998;17:283–295.

34. Mullahy J. Much ado about two: reconsidering retransformation and the two-part model in health econometrics. *J Health Econ.* 1998;17:247–281.

35. Manning WG, Mullahy J. Estimating log models: to transform or not to transform. *J Health Econ.* 2001;20:461–494.

36. Thompson SG, Barber JA. How should cost data in pragmatic randomized trials be analysed? *Br Med J.* 2000;320:1197–1200.

37. Basu A, Manning WG, Mullahy J. Comparing alternative models: log vs proportional hazard? *Health Econ.* 2004;13:749–765.

38. Deb P and Trivedi PK. The structure of demand for health care: latent class versus two-part models. *J Health Econ.* 2002;21:601–625.

39. Lin DY, Feuer EJ, Etzioni R, Wax Y. Estimating medical costs from incomplete follow-up. *Biometrics.* 1997;53:419–434.

40. Bang H, Tsiatis AA. Estimating medical costs with censored data. *Biometrika.* 2000;87:329–343.

41. Lin DY. Linear regression analysis of censored medical costs. *Biostatistics.* 2000;1:35–47.

42. Lin DY. Proportional means regression for censored medical costs. *Biometrics.* 2000;56:775–778.

43. Zhao H, Tian L. On estimating medical cost and incremental cost-effectiveness ratios with censored data. *Biometrics.* 2001;57:1002–1008.

44. Willan AR, Lin DY, Cook RJ, Chen EB. Using inverse-weighting in cost-effectiveness analysis with censored data. *Stat Methods Med Res.* 2002;11:539–551.

45. O'Hagan A, Stevens JW. On estimators of medical costs with censored data. *J Health Econ.* 2004;23:615–625.

46. Jain AK, Strawderman RL. Flexible hazard regression modeling for medical cost data. *Biostatistics.* 2002;3:101–118.

47. Baser O, Gardiner JC, Bradley CJ, Given CW. Estimation from censored medical cost data. *Biometrical Journal,* 2004;46(1):351–363.

48. Curtis LH, Hammill BG, Eisenstein EL, Kramer JM, Anstrom KJ. Using inverse probability-weighted estimators in comparative effectiveness analyses with observational databases. *Medical Care.* 2007;45:S103–S107.

49. Efron B, Ribshirani R. *An Introduction to the Bootstrap.* New York, NY: Chapman & Hall, 1993.

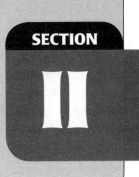
Evaluating Levels of Evidence

Chapter 6 explores the randomized controlled trial (RCT), one of the most common and strongest research designs available. The RCT typically focuses on answering a research question, such as why one solution (a drug or intervention approach) is better (superiority trials) or no different than (noninferiority clinical trials) another solution. The US Food and Drug Administration (FDA) requires pharmaceutical companies to conduct clinical trials involving RCTs to demonstrate the efficacy and safety of their drug before a drug can be marketed and sold. In addition to study designs and sample size selection, the overall generalizability of a study is key, because this will impact how the study results will be interpreted and used in the general population of interest. Lastly, for a study to be humane and ethical, clinical researchers must take responsibility to protect participants from harm and follow procedures such as obtaining institutional review board approval and informed consent from study subjects before the study begins and patients are enrolled, respectively.

As described in Chapter 7, systematic reviews and meta-analyses make valuable contributions to the literature of assessment because they have the potential to forcefully summarize the magnitude of treatment effects, when individual studies leave the question(s) unresolved. Both systematic reviews and meta-analyses can help guide clinical decision making until large trials can be completed, but neither is a substitute for large clinical trials. They also have the potential to assist in the development of treatment guidelines. Like any clinical trial, there are rigorous techniques for conducting both systematic reviews and meta-analyses, including eligibility criteria of articles defined a priori.

Although RCTs are the accepted "gold standard" for determining cause and effect of medical interventions, they cannot be conducted in all situations, such as when they are either unethical or cost prohibitive to conduct. One alternative is to conduct research using existing secondary data sources such as medical and prescription claims databases. Chapter 8 discusses the advantages and disadvantages of using these types of claims data and the types of studies that can be undertaken using these data. Furthermore, practical information on sources of claims data and how to conduct a study using claims data is provided.

This section concludes with Chapter 9, a chapter devoted to a growing area of studies that include some aspect of patient-reported outcomes within them. In addition, the use of patient registries and observational databases, as well as other sources of patient data such as electronic health records, is described. In some instances, these data may be referred to as "real-world data" because they do not come directly from RCTs.

Randomized Controlled Trials

Nathaniel M. Rickles, PharmD, PhD, BCPP
Matthew Wolfe, BA

Learning Objectives

- Identify the use of randomized controlled trials (RCTs) in drug use research.
- Compare and contrast the advantages and disadvantages of RCTs.
- Describe key considerations in selecting participants and developing study protocols.
- Distinguish between the different types of study outcomes.
- Determine ways to monitor RCT implementation.
- Differentiate ways to analyze study data and how they affect study outcomes.
- Describe different limitations that can affect the application of study findings.

■ Introduction

There are many research designs one can employ to study different research questions. For example, a researcher interested in obtaining a description of a problem might consider using an observational study design that involves simple data collection and the reporting of findings. In this chapter, we will explore one of the strongest research designs available, the *randomized controlled trial* (*RCT*), to answer research questions focused on why one solution (a drug or intervention approach) is better (superiority trials) or no different than another solution (noninferiority clinical trials). Within the health care community, randomized controlled designs are often used to scientifically compare the effectiveness of one drug with another drug and/or placebo. Before a drug can be marketed and sold, the US Food and Drug Administration (FDA) requires pharmaceutical companies to conduct clinical RCTs to demonstrate the efficacy and safety of their drug.

What makes the RCT a strong research design? The RCT allows the researcher to control for factors and biases that can confound the true effect of an intervention. Other research designs are not as well controlled, and therefore, various factors can affect the relationships being explored. The following example might help clarify the value of the RCT over other designs. A researcher wants to explore whether Drug A is an effective treatment for depression. She decides to set up a *prospective cohort study* by identifying a sample of depressed individuals who are being treated with Drug A and observing how Drug A affects the population sample at some point in the future. Alternatively, she can set up a *retrospective cohort study* that identifies a cohort of depressed individuals treated with Drug A in the past and examines what their outcomes are at present.

The researcher is left with many questions from both of these designs. Do the samples have any characteristics that can affect outcomes, such as severity of illness and the type of practice settings in which the participants receive treatment? Are there any intervening factors that may have contributed to the outcomes outside of Drug A? Do we know whether administering Drug A is more effective than giving the participants a different drug or a placebo (sugar pill)? Did researchers and/or prescribers affect outcomes because they knew the participants who received Drug A? These unanswered questions cast doubt on any findings from these studies that Drug A is effective in the treatment of depression. As will be discussed in this chapter, an RCT helps to answer these questions and provide greater confidence in the findings of studies.

Several examples exist of important RCTs from over the last decade or so that have influenced clinical decision making. RCTs from the Women's Health Initiative (WHI) investigated whether conjugated equine estrogen alone or in combination with progestin would reduce cardiovascular events in healthy postmenopausal women with prior hysterectomies.[1] The WHI trial examining the combination of estrogen and progestin was halted due to concern that the risks exceeded the benefits. The researchers found that coronary heart disease, stroke, and other cardiovascular syndromes increased more in participants who received combination therapy than in the controls. They also noted that the combination therapy was associated with an increase in incidence of breast cancer but a decrease in risk for hip fractures. Another WHI study showed that estrogens alone increased the risk of strokes and decreased the risk of hip fracture with no change in the incidence of cardiovascular heart disease.[2] The authors found the incidence of disease to be similar across the estrogen and placebo groups. Such findings led the authors to conclude that estrogen should not be recommended for chronic disease prevention in postmenopausal women. These WHI studies were widely publicized and led women to question the risks and benefits of hormone replacement therapy.

Having considered the overall value and examples of RCTs, we will now shift to discussing specific aspects of how to set up an RCT, issues involved in implementation, considerations in evaluation, and interpretation of findings. As we proceed through these next sections, it is helpful to think about a specific study we might want to perform. Let's say we are interested in evaluating the impact of a Web-based antidepressant self-monitoring program on participant outcomes such as antidepressant adherence, participant satisfaction, and participant self-efficacy in treatment. Where would we start and why?

■ Development of an RCT

The first step in developing an RCT is to conduct a literature review and find out what research designs have been used in the past so that we can avoid duplication and benefit from the experiences of other trials. Let's say that our literature review yields several study types: a cross-sectional study and several prospective and retrospective cohort studies of participant self-management of depression. The cross-sectional study involved a report on a past survey administered to a group of participants with depression who completed online diaries of their symptoms. This study found participants reporting significant satisfaction with self-tracking symptoms using a diary method.

The cohort studies, however, yielded mixed findings. In the prospective cohort study, the researchers followed a group of participants who used a weekly symptom checklist to monitor their depression symptoms. They found that the checklist was not associated with greater feelings of self-control of illness. In the retrospective cohort study, the researchers used data from a large study collected over the previous 2 years by a managed care organization that tracked symptoms and side effects reported by participants using an online tool. These latter researchers found that the online tool yielded significant improvement in antidepressant adherence. As indicated earlier, however, these study designs do not tell us whether Web-based self-monitoring contributed to improved outcomes. For example, were reported findings due to how the study population was selected and other variables that could have contributed to the outcomes? We need to tease out some of these possible explanations for the mixed results and see whether a study under controlled conditions would yield different results. Therefore, we decide to perform an RCT.

Selection of Study Participants

RCTs typically aim to compare how 2 or more groups respond to 1 or more treatment approaches. One or more of the study groups involve participants who are actively receiving a treatment approach (known as the *intervention group*). Another comparison group includes those who have not received any treatment approaches or have received the standard treatment approach that exists in practice, that is, usual care (known as the *control group*). In an RCT involving medications, the researcher may use a *placebo* in the control group as a means of appearing to provide an active treatment while in fact providing none. Placebo pills will look very similar or identical to active medication but contain no active medication. The advantage of using placebos is that participants will not know whether or not they received the medication and thus will not be biased in reporting efficacy or toxicities.

The scientific community has raised recent concerns that many trials report positive therapeutic findings among participants who use placebos and such positive effects affect the significance of study findings.[3] There has been considerable discussion as to why participants are reporting such positive results using a therapeutically inactive product (eg, a placebo capsule or pill).[4,5] It is possible that these positive placebo results are caused by (1) participants wanting to please the researcher and report favorable results, (2) participants feeling a need to justify taking a pill by indicating that it has positive effects (otherwise it would not make sense to continue taking the pill), (3) participants reporting positive effects because they feel they are being observed and cared for by being in the study, and (4) participants feeling better when not on a medication that may have had negative side effects or made them feel worse.

An RCT can involve comparing multiple treatment approaches or intervention groups with control groups. What the researchers decide to compare is largely determined by the research question being addressed. When exposure to the intervention and control groups occurs at the same time, such a research model is often referred to as a *parallel design*. Because our research question wishes to examine whether a Web-based antidepressant self-monitoring program is better than what participants currently do to self-monitor their antidepressant use, we will have 2 groups: an intervention group in which participants will be asked to use a Web-based self-monitoring antidepressant program and a control group in which participants will be expected to self-monitor their antidepressant treatment as they typically would ("usual care approach").

In contrast to a parallel design, researchers might use a *crossover research design* that does not involve the study of 2 separate parallel groups. This design exposes the same participants to both study groups over time. In this way, the participants serve as their own controls. For example, a participant might be assigned to receive the treatment for 6 weeks and then be switched to receive usual care for the next 6 weeks. Researchers would examine differences in participant outcomes after completing each 6 weeks.

Once we know what groups of participants we will have, we have to think carefully regarding the kind of people who will be in both groups. RCTs typically do this by setting clear *inclusion and exclusion criteria* about who should and should not be included in the study. These selection criteria establish a set of conditions that participants must meet at baseline so that researchers have the best chance of clearly identifying the impact of the intervention on the target participant population. To find results that are clinically relevant to the treatment's anticipated outcome, a trial will need to have participants who are at greatest risk for a negative outcome if not treated.[6] The most basic inclusion criterion is the target condition. A pharmaceutical company testing a new drug for attention deficit disorder (ADD) would want participants who have been diagnosed with ADD. Perhaps the focus is on adults; so a diagnosis of ADD and an age of 18 years or older would be inclusion criteria. Other possible inclusion criteria might involve race, sex, stage of illness, and income.

In the ADD study, baseline characteristics such as other cognitive disorders might confound results. As a result, prior head trauma or past use of certain illicit substances might be used as exclusion criteria. Researchers conducting RCTs will often choose to exclude complex participants with multiple disease states or with prior experiences with the intervention to avoid factors that might affect study conclusions or when there may be safety issues associated with their participation. Clinical trials often exclude participants who are more susceptible to potential or known harmful adverse effects due to preexisting conditions or interactions with other drugs.[6] Researchers might also exclude participants who are unlikely to complete the intervention (eg, people with transportation difficulties, language barriers, illiteracy, and other disabilities deemed to limit involvement).

RCTs should clearly state the inclusion and exclusion criteria. Although the use of multiple inclusion and exclusion criteria helps isolate a clear population to benefit from the study, it may also make recruitment difficult. Sometimes researchers have to modify their selection criteria to obtain a sufficient number of participants prior to the initiation of the study. Changing the selection criteria during an ongoing study might pose some concerns of selection bias because participants entering the study before the change may be different than participants entering the study after the selection criteria have changed.[7] These changes can possibly contribute to differences in study outcomes.

Researchers will often try to statistically control in their data analysis for some of the factors of participants they allowed to enter the study by opening the study to involve more participants. There has been also considerable concern with RCTs having so many inclusion and exclusion criteria that the study groups do not reflect the real-world participant population. The very effort of avoiding confounding variables by setting several inclusion and exclusion criteria may affect how applicable study results are to participants seen in everyday practice. The extent to which a study population reflects the typical population is known as *generalizability*. Most researchers will note any generalizability concerns in the limitations discussion of the final published report.

In our study of Web-based self-monitoring of antidepressant therapy, we will exclude the following: (1) individuals less than 18 years old, (2) those who do not have consistent access and knowledge of how to use computers, (3) those who cannot read and understand English, and (4) those currently using a self-monitoring approach to assess antidepressant therapy. We exclude those less than 18 years old because the developed Web-based tool is best suited for adults and may require changes when used for children and teenagers. The second and third criteria are included because the Web-based monitoring program requires knowledge of how to use computers and understand the English-based tools. By setting the fourth criteria, we avoid the confounding effect of dual exposure to more than one self-monitoring program. With such dual exposure, it would be hard to distinguish whether study findings are due to the Web-based monitoring program, some other self-monitoring program, or both programs.

Determination of Sample Size

Determining sample size for a study requires careful consideration of various factors such as the study design, desired effect size, type of statistical test being used, probability of finding a difference in study groups when in reality there is none (called a *type I error* or α *error*), and probability of not finding a difference when one exists (*type II error* or

β *error*). A study design that involves 2 parallel groups will require a different number of participants to detect differences between participants than a design that explores differences within participants (such as the crossover design). *Effect size* is a number that reflects the extent to which the study will be able to detect the effects of the intervention on the study outcome. This number is not always easy to determine and is often arbitrary.

Sometimes past literature is useful in describing what would be considered a significant clinical and/or statistical difference in the outcomes measured. For example, if we want to see if Web-based self-monitoring of antidepressant therapy improves participant satisfaction, what does the past literature report as a significant difference in participant satisfaction across 2 groups? If our research informs us that we only need to detect large differences in participant satisfaction to find significant results, then we may need to enroll a smaller number of participants. However, if we learn that only small differences in participant satisfaction are significant, we may need to enroll much larger samples to detect those differences.

To test different hypotheses, a researcher will use different statistical tests depending on the type of data (continuous, dichotomous) and the level of analysis (bivariate, multivariate). Different numbers of participants are needed to detect differences using different statistical tests. Researchers can also establish different criteria for detecting type I or II errors. When researchers determine that they are willing to accept a 5% chance that a type I error will occur, they set the level of significance (α) at .05. In other words, the researchers are saying that there is a 95% chance that they are not committing a type I error. In general, most researchers set α at .05. The more stringent the α level, such as .01 or .001, the more difficult it is to find a statistical difference. Many more participants are likely to be needed if the α is made more stringent. In a similar fashion, if a researcher sets the β at .10, then the investigator is willing to accept a 10% chance of reporting no difference when one exists (type II error). The more we want to avoid a type II error, the more participants the researchers will need to include in the study.

Often RCTs involve the calculation of *power*, which is the probability of detecting a treatment difference when one exists. Most RCTs aim for a power of at least 80% or allow that there is a 20% chance of finding there is no difference when one truly exists. When reporting power, it is important to state what the difference is that the power analysis was calculated to detect. For example, a researcher might indicate that to obtain 80% power, 200 participants are needed to detect a difference of 20% in medication adherence between the intervention and control groups. One way to improve the power of a study or the chance of finding a difference when one exists is to increase the number of participants in the study. It should also be noted that sample size/power analysis is often calculated based on the primary study end point, but researchers can also calculate power based on secondary end points and adjust the sample size so that they can find a statistical difference for all outcomes of interest.

In addition to the previously mentioned considerations in determining sample size, researchers also need to consider attrition issues when determining how many participants to enroll. If researchers expect to lose a certain percentage of participants, they should increase their target sample size at the beginning of the study by that percentage. By anticipating attrition, the researchers can achieve the sample size needed to detect the statistical differences they expect to find.

In our Web-based antidepressant self-monitoring study, we find literature indicating that Web-based interventions have produced medium to large effect sizes of 70%. At a conventional power of 80% and α of .05, and using t tests for means, Cohen's power tables indicate a sample size of 26 participants per intervention group and control group.[8] To allow for at least 20% attrition and achieve a power of at least 80%, we decided to recruit 80 participants (40 participants in each of the study groups).

Recruitment of Study Participants

Many researchers openly report the difficulty of recruiting participants for studies. It is often difficult to stimulate participant interest in research. Potential participants often struggle with such issues as whether they have time for the study, their comfort with experimental procedures, and general concern about the use of any of their health information. Investigators are often at task to generate interest through creative announcements, financial incentives, and/or expectation that they will benefit science in some meaningful way. The researcher needs to be careful as to what an appropriate incentive might be because too much of an incentive might seem coercive and too little may not sufficiently motivate the potential participant. Researchers should allow sufficient time for enrollment because enrollment can often take considerably longer than expected. It should also be noted that recruitment may differ during different times of the year, with holidays and summers being more difficult as a result of vacations.

Assignment of Study Participants

Once the research team has identified participants who meet the study's inclusion and exclusion criteria and how many participants they need, the team will then seek to assign the participants to treatment and/or control groups. Why are participants not assigned based on their desire to be in a particular group or based on a clinician's preference for which group the participants get assigned to? If this occurs, the researcher worries that there is some extraneous factor associated with self-selection or clinician selection that may differentially affect how participants respond to their exposure to treatment or usual care.

For example, physicians may decide they want participants who are less independent and have poorer control of their depression to be in the Web-based self-monitoring group and participants who are more independent in the usual care group. Such a selection decision may produce a disproportionate number of poorly controlled individuals in the intervention group. As a result, the researchers may find the Web-based monitoring to be less effective than usual care when in fact it may have little to do with the intervention but with the clinical severity of the participants in the group.

Likewise, if participants self-selects into the intervention group, they may be more likely to be actively engaged in treatment and bias the results toward the efficacy of the intervention. Both participant self-selection and clinician selection are issues associated with *selection bias*. Selection bias occurs when study participants are assigned differentially to a study group due to a variable outside of the inclusion criteria. As noted in the previous examples, this variable can contribute to differential outcomes.

How do we help avoid selection bias and improve generalizability? We randomly assign participants to a study group. *Randomization* is a process by which each study participant has an equal probability of being assigned to study groups. Researchers use many techniques to randomize participants. Some of these include (1) use of a random number generator available in many software programs, (2) random number tables commonly available in statistics books, and (3) randomly selecting study identification numbers and establishing before the study begins which study group the identification number is associated with. This technique of randomization is commonly used with phase II and III clinical trials.[6] Randomization helps to reduce selection bias because participants have equal probability of being assigned to a group.

The randomization process also helps to improve generalizability because random assignment allows the participants with a variety of factors (which could confound results) to be equally assigned to a study group. As such, participants associated with various possible confounding factors (such as age, sex, and education level) have an equal chance of being in any study group. This allows the study groups to better represent the typical participant population because medical practices see participants with varying background characteristics. Researchers will often report in their research reports the extent to which study groups were similar to the characteristics of the typical participant population served by the treatment approach and how similar study groups were to each other. If baseline characteristics of study groups are significantly different from those of the typical participant population, study results may not be very generalizable. If study groups are significantly different from each other on certain key factors, then the differences could contribute to differences in study findings. If either of these latter situations occurred, they should be noted as potential limitations.

Methods exist for making distribution more even, particularly in trials with smaller numbers of participants. The first technique, *block randomization*, is commonly used to ensure that the number of participants is equally distributed among study groups. Randomization is done within blocks of predetermined size.[6] This means that in a study involving 30 participants assigned to 2 groups, randomization can be set to occur within 2 separate groups of 15. Researchers can also make randomization less predictable by varying the size of each group within a range (eg, 13 to 17 participants).

Stratified block randomization (also known as *restricted randomization*) is used to ensure that similar numbers of people with different characteristics, usually those that can be predictors of the outcome, are assigned to each group and that the distribution of baseline variables is more equal. This can be done by dividing the study cohort into 2 groups, each one with or without a certain characteristic, and then carrying out a block randomization within each "strata." This method minimizes the disparity between groups by taking into account a variety of variables. Stratified block randomization is also valuable when there are known proportions of participants in a population and the researchers desire to achieve similar proportions in their sample (so the study sample resembles the population).[6] For example, if a researcher knows that a particular medication is used by 65% of African Americans, 25% of Caucasians, and 10% of Asians and is conducting a study involving this medication among 100 participants, then the researcher might want to stratify the sample by randomly assigning 65 African Americans, 25 Caucasians, and 10 Asians to the intervention and/or control groups. One concern with this approach is that the last assigned person in a block is essentially predetermined. Additionally, balancing treatment groups by means of an allocation scheme undermines true randomization. Despite these drawbacks, these methods help allow for some randomization but yet best reflect the target population.

Although randomization reduces selection bias and improves generalizability, it can do little to prevent bias that occurs during follow-up.[6] Such biases can occur if clinicians are aware of the participants' group assignments, leading to differences in treatment between groups and influencing the clinician's assessment of outcomes. For example, if a participant knows he is in the intervention group and expects the intervention to yield better outcomes, he may report more favorable outcomes than if he had been in the control group. The same concern holds for the investigator who expects certain outcomes and biases the intervention and/or analysis to yield those outcomes (known as *ascertainment bias*).[6] One important way to reduce such biases in follow-up is known as *blinding*. In a study that involves blinding, the participants and/or investigators do not know whether the participants are in the intervention or control groups. Specifically, a study that involves blinding of only the participant and not the investigator is considered *single blinded*. A study in which the participant and the investigator are blinded is considered *double blinded*.

Blinding can be difficult to carry out and maintain. Blinding associated with a drug therapy trial will involve the masking of the placebo or other treatment arm so the participant and physician/researcher cannot recognize the medicine by sight, smell, or touch. The manufacturer or pharmacy will construct a placebo or active treatment to look and feel identical to the comparison treatment. If participants become sick possibly due to adverse events, unblinding can be avoided by directing them to a physician with no involvement in the study. A good way to assess the effectiveness and success of blinding and to check for potential bias is to ask the participants and the investigators after the study is over to guess the treatment assignments.[6]

If there appears to be significant complications in one treatment arm over the other, an investigator may have to stop the trial and remove blinding to discover which intervention is causing the complications. Blinding is often difficult to accomplish in many

RCTs investigating the value of services provided to individuals because it is difficult to keep the identity of intervention and control groups unknown to participants and investigators. Thus, it is difficult to involve blinding in our Web-based antidepressant self-monitoring study because both the participant and the investigator are aware of the participant's use of a Web-based antidepressant self-monitoring program.

■ Consent and Ethical Considerations

Any study that involves human participants should adhere to a certain standard of ethics. Today, ethics consist of generally accepted rules of moral conduct that have been codified by the medical community. They are especially important to RCTs with human participants. The purpose of clinical research is the advancement of scientific knowledge for the benefit of humanity, but the well-being of study participants must be safeguarded as well. There are several main principles of bioethics: beneficence (doing the right thing), nonmaleficence (doing no harm), respect for the individual's autonomy, fidelity (being faithful and keeping a promise), veracity (being truthful), and justice.[9,10] Experiments can expose participants to risk, so beneficence must be central to any clinical study. When research unintentionally or willfully disregards the well-being of human participants, however, the noble pursuit of scientific knowledge is compromised. For a study to be humane and ethical, clinical researchers must take responsibility to protect participants from harm. Laws and guidelines dictating proper ethical research with human participants were developed during the second half of the 20th century in reaction to the uncovering of instances of severe misconduct in research.

During World War II, Nazi physicians conducted torturous medical experiments on Jewish people, prisoners of war, the disabled, the malformed, and other "unfit" inmates of concentration camps against their will. The experiments included placing people in freezing water to study hypothermia, subjecting them to dramatic changes in atmospheric pressure, exposing them to poison gases, deliberate infection with lethal germs, sterilization, and other painful procedures carried out against the will of the participants. The purpose of the experiments was often to study the hazards encountered by soldiers and pilots in battle, but Nazi physicians also toyed with human bodies seemingly to satisfy their own morbid curiosities. Although some prisoners were killed before undergoing such torturous experimentation, many others were forced to endure painful procedures without anesthetic. Also during this time, Japanese researchers killed thousands of Chinese people in similar forced medical experiments.[9]

Following the war, the revelation of the Nazis' cruel experimentation on human beings made it clear that there needed to be a body of rules governing human experimentation. The first attempt at curbing medical research performed via coercive or other unethical means was the Nuremberg Code written in 1947 during the Nuremberg Trials. Consisting of 10 points, it included such important principles as informed consent, avoidance of harm to participants, and proper ethical considerations for running a clinical trial. The World Medical Association, also formed in 1947, first drafted the Declaration of Helsinki in 1964. The Declaration of Helsinki are guidelines involving ethical principles for medical research that includes human subjects, identifiable human material and data.

The Tuskegee syphilis study is another historical example of how researchers have been unethical. In 1932, researchers began a prospective clinical trial to observe the progression of syphilis in African American males in Macon County, Alabama. At that time, because penicillin had not yet been discovered as a cure for syphilis, clinicians were not depriving participants of the most effective treatment, because there was none available. By the 1940s, however, penicillin was already the standard for treatment of the disease, and Tuskegee researchers not only denied participants access to it, but also actively prevented them from receiving the proper treatment. Moreover, the study recruited mostly illiterate African American sharecroppers infected with the disease and attracted them with misleading announcements, ensuring that they were unaware of their disease's progression and denial of treatment. At the study's end in 1972, most of the original test participants had died, 40 of their wives had been infected, and 19 children were born with congenital syphilis.[11]

The Tuskegee experiment remains one of the most disturbing episodes in American medical history. What began as an experiment intended to benefit the health of America's poor population soon became an observational study in which people were mere objects to be observed while denied the benefits of modern medicine. Despite this unfortunate episode, experts have drawn on this experience to further shape ethical policies that ensure the most proper humane treatment of people who participate in scientific research. With research abuses taking place such as the Tuskegee syphilis study, the Declaration of Helsinki has been revised 6 times. The 1975 revision introduced the concept of institutional review (discussed in the following paragraph), which soon became part of US law.

Today, rules on medical ethics mandate that clinicians may only enroll participants who are fully aware of what they are getting involved with and have agreed to participate (known as *informed consent*). For the consent to be valid, participants must be made aware of all benefits and risks relevant to the study in a language that they understand, and they must also have the capacity to understand and make decisions to participate in the study or not. All trials in the United States are required to participate with independent ethical review boards to ensure that proper procedures are followed. This independent review process is carried out by an *institutional review board* (IRB), which is required by the National Institutes of Health and other agencies to monitor and approve clinical study protocols in order for the study to receive funding. The IRB reviews protocols and informed consent documents, making sure that the consent document is written in a way that is easy to read and understand and details all the necessary information for a consumer to make an appropriate decision.[9] TABLE 6-1 provides information regarding key components of what belongs in a typical consent form. Funding agencies will require all research involving human participants to be approved by the IRB prior to the initiation of any aspects of the study.

Table 6-1	Interactive Informed Consent Template

What is the purpose of this form and reason for the informed consent process?

Information must be comprehensible and understood fully by the participant.

Indicate that questions are allowed for further clarification.

Participant has the authority to deny or agree to participate

What is the purpose of the study?

Explain briefly and concisely why the study is being conducted.

Why is it important to participate?

Explain the value of the study and how results will help participant and others.

What will the participant's role be?

Describe tasks of participant.

Detail what participant may experience (ie, explain procedures).

What are conditions of participation and withdrawal?

Participation is voluntary.

Refusal or withdrawal from study will not result in penalty.

What extent of confidentiality does the participant have?

Explain who will have access to data.

Data may contain patient identity or be blinded data.

What foreseeable risks, harms, discomfort, or inconvenience may the participant experience? Or state none, if applicable.

Indicate likelihood and seriousness of risk or harm.

Indicate precautions to minimize risk or harm.

Are there any benefits to the participant?

Describe any direct benefits the participant will receive as a result of study involvement (this does not include financial incentives).

How much time will the participant need to commit to?

Indicate how much time each part of the participant's work will take.

What alternatives are there to the research protocol?

Note any other options available besides study participation through which the participant can receive similar treatment or services as in the study.

Will there be any compensation for participation?

May include injury compensation, if applicable.

Who can the participant contact if questions arise regarding the study or the participant's rights or in case of injury?

Provide contact information of study coordinator for study questions/injuries and institutional review board regarding participant rights.

Is there any other pertinent information that may not be stated elsewhere?

Age requirement.

Address vulnerable populations (pregnant women, children, prisoners, and mentally impaired).

Source: Data from National Institutes of Health, Office of Extramural Research. Protecting human research participants. http://phrp.nihtraining.com/index.php. Accessed October 29, 2009; and Northeastern University, Office of Human Subject Research Protection. Human subjects research forms and instructions (IRB). http://www.northeastern.edu/research/facts_rates_forms/forms/#human_forms. Accessed October 29, 2009.

Involving a person in medical research is a serious matter that is not taken lightly. Trials of treatments that are not fully proven can have a potential risk of harm, use much funding, and be physically draining on participants. Thus a study is only ethical if it has a reasonable likelihood of producing intended answer(s) to the research question(s) posed. Additionally, it is wasteful to continue a trial after a question has already been answered.

Clinical trials are run with the intention of finding an answer to a research question. Once an answer has been found, there is no need to continue a trial. Federal and other funding agencies often require a *data and safety monitoring board* that will periodically evaluate study findings for safety and effectiveness. Researchers may decide to prematurely end a trial because (1) the harm of an intervention outweighs the benefit and/or (2) there is a clear benefit shown in one study group and not others. It is important to bear in mind that once a trial is stopped, the chance to find more conclusive results and information is lost. When deciding whether to stop a trial, researchers must weigh their duty to advance scientific knowledge against their ethical responsibility to keep participants safe.

In the early 1970s, researchers at Smith, Kline & French were testing an H_2-receptor antagonist, metiamide, in participants with duodenal ulcer. They took participants off the drug immediately when it was found that the drug was causing agranulocytosis, or decreased white blood cell counts, leaving participants susceptible to infection. The researchers learned that it was a particular chemical moiety associated with metiamide's chemistry that contributed to the agranulocytosis. After removing this chemical moiety, the new chemical compound, cimetidine, was deemed safe and effective for treating and preventing ulcers. Cimetidine went on to become a very popular prescription and, later, over-the-counter medication to reduce stomach acid and prevent and treat ulcers.[12]

Clinicians have the ethical responsibility to offer participants the best, most effective available treatment. Randomizing participants to a therapy or a placebo, however, presents a major ethical dilemma. By administering one intervention over another to participants, researchers may be denying the control group a more effective therapy. **Equipoise,** or indifference toward the relative merits of 2 or more different treatments, somewhat resolves this issue by suggesting that a researcher is free of this responsibility if he or she has no clear evidence that one treatment is superior to another.[7] Studies that compare 2 equally effective treatments are called *noninferiority trials*. Such trials avoid the ethical conflict of randomly assigning participants in need of medication to a placebo arm. Noninferiority study designs are often used for anti-infective medications (eg, antibiotics, antivirals).

It is also unethical to discourage or prohibit participants from taking other treatments that may be of important benefit to them.[6] Participants should be made aware in the consent form that there are other options available to them outside of the interventions associated with the study. In our Web-based antidepressant self-monitoring study, we will submit our study procedures and consent form for review to an IRB.

■ RCT Implementation

One of the most important aspects to carefully think about when developing an RCT are the steps involved in the RCT implementation phase. A poorly conceived implementation can contribute to unclear findings. The intervention should be as structured as possible so results can be clearly tied to the intervention and not other aspects. Furthermore, the more structured and clear the description of the intervention, the easier it is for researchers to replicate the intervention. Essentially, the description of the intervention should answer all the basic questions of who, what, where, when, why, and how.

Researchers should clearly identify who will administer the intervention and any training they will receive to provide the intervention. Ideally, the researcher should include some way to assess *program fidelity*. Program fidelity is a term that refers to a researcher's effort to make sure the intervention was carried out systematically and consistently as planned. For example, researchers might design a checklist that those carrying out the intervention need to use to document that they performed certain intervention tasks. If a researcher can have a high degree of confidence that the intervention was carried out as planned, then she can have greater confidence that the outcomes are associated with the intervention and not some modification of it. Interestingly, many research papers omit any documentation of program fidelity, which complicates the interpretation of findings. If a control group is used, it should be clear how this group will not be exposed to the intervention. The length of the intervention and when outcomes will be collected should be clearly described. To assess program fidelity in our Web-based antidepressant self-monitoring study, we will collect user statistics of the Web pages. We will examine how often participants went to the Web site to report their symptoms and side effects. Did they go to the Web site at least once a month as expected?

Researchers can take several measures to maximize adherence to the study protocol and minimize dropout. First, the intervention should be administered to participants as soon as possible following randomization. The longer the time between randomization and the active treatment, the more likely there will be participants who drop out early without receiving their assigned intervention.[13] Second, care should be taken to ensure that follow-up visits are personable, not stressful, and enjoyable. Third, researchers can also make participants feel more involved by informing them of the importance of follow-up and showing them results.

Prestudy phases can be used to exclude participants who are unlikely to contribute to the main outcome. One simple way to do this is by asking participants to make 1 or 2 screening visits to the clinic before randomization. Screening visits allow investigators to exclude participants who are incapable of making such visits prior to the actual study. To most closely represent the actual likelihood of participants to follow protocol, screening visits should not be too easy for participants to make, but they should not be so difficult that participants lose motivation or interest in the study.[6]

In addition, researchers might want to use a "run-in period" that provides a few weeks of no treatment (placebo) to test the participant's adherence to study protocol. Then, after a period of a few weeks, participants who prove to be adherent can be randomized to the active treatment or to continue the placebo, whereas nonadherent participants can be excluded from the study. A "run-in period" also allows researchers to wean participants off other therapies that conflict with study protocol. This extra study period does prolong the study and may use up additional time, money, and energy but, in the long run, may provide greater return by reducing participant dropouts.

The sequencing of the intervention with outcome measures is important because the researcher wants to capture the direct effects of different phases of the intervention or the lack of an intervention. Researchers may want to involve multiple data collections of outcome measures so they can observe patterns. When possible, it is recommended that researchers use previously described and validated measures. Such validated measures give the researcher greater confidence that outcomes are more related to the intervention than issues with measurement. It is not always possible to use existing measures because none may exist for a variety of topics. If new measures are being used, researchers should report the results of any validation testing of instruments done prior to study implementation.

Careful attention should also be paid to how the outcomes are collected. Researchers can bias their own data collection by making participants aware of their presence (often known as the *Hawthorne Effect*). An example of this occurs with *surveillance bias*. Surveillance bias occurs when one study group is followed more closely than another group and this differentially affects study outcomes. One way to reduce surveillance bias is by researchers collecting outcomes for all study groups at the same time periods. Another example of how researchers can impact study outcomes is through *interviewer bias*. This bias occurs during face-to-face data collection; different interviewers ask questions differently, and this contributes to differences in responses/outcomes. If a study does not involve blinding, the researcher may ask intervention participants questions differently than control participants based on their desired outcomes. Blinding group assignment helps reduce the likelihood of such bias.

Researchers should also be aware of other biases that can affect data collection and the validity of their outcome measures. Participants may respond to questions (especially sensitive ones) by telling researchers what they want to hear and not truly how they feel. This type of bias is called *social desirability bias*. Several ways to reduce social desirability bias are by making outcome measures anonymous and providing a brief statement before asking the sensitive questions that makes any response socially acceptable and consistent with what others might do. In most cases, it may be difficult to keep outcome data completely anonymous because researchers need to link outcome data back to the participant. However, the researcher can identify the participant with a study identification number that is indicated on all outcome measures collected. This way, the outcome measures are not identifiable in themselves but, when needed, can be linked to a list kept separately of participants and their study identification numbers.

Two additional considerations for researchers when determining their outcome measures are *recall bias* and *respondent burden*. Recall bias occurs when participants have difficulty recalling certain information. Most commonly, participants have difficulty recalling past events and behaviors that occurred awhile ago versus events and behaviors that occurred recently. Such difficulty in recall may affect the validity of what is being recalled. It is generally recommended to keep the recall period as short as possible to avoid errors in recall. Respondent burden indicates all the tasks and time that researchers ask a participant to do and give for participation. The more tasks that are requested, the greater the respondent burden and the more likely the participant will have difficulty completing the tasks or decide to withdraw from the study. Long surveys can also increase respondent burden; researchers should try to limit surveys to the absolute number of items to obtain the data needed to answer their research questions.

In the Web-based antidepressant monitoring project, we will collect several outcome measures for all study participants (intervention and control) over the study period. Data will be collected at the baseline, midpoint, and end of the study period so we can see how outcomes vary across the time period. As identified earlier, we will examine 3 primary outcomes: antidepressant adherence, participant satisfaction, and participant self-efficacy. We will ask all participants to complete brief self-administered surveys that ask items that self-report their antidepressant adherence over a 7-day reference period, satisfaction, and self-efficacy at baseline, midpoint, and the end of the study. We will use existing measures of self-reported medication adherence and modify existing measures for treatment satisfaction and self-efficacy. Because self-reports of adherence may be influenced by social desirability bias, we will also collect pharmacy refill records over the study period to objectively assess antidepressant adherence at baseline, midpoint, and the end of the study period.

■ RCT Analysis and Evaluation

The aim of the data collection efforts identified in the previous section on RCT implementation is to yield valid data from all study participants throughout the entire study period. Such valid data can then be analyzed to test study hypotheses and answer related research questions. The present section will present reasons why researchers may not have valid data for all study participants and how researchers can adjust their analyses for such losses when interpreting the results.

Common reasons for why participants may need to officially withdraw from a study may include the following: participant experiences adverse events; participant develops a condition during the study that causes the participant to be unable to remain in the study; participant enrolls in another trial and researcher needs to avoid confounding results; and participant moves away or dies. Participants may never tell researchers their intention to not complete all outcome measures due to a lack of interest or being too busy.

Loss to follow-up can result in biased results and undermine the statistical power of a study (researchers did not achieve the sample size needed to detect a significance difference in their results). Loss to follow-up can especially skew results if the very cause of discontinuation, such as a side effect or lack of efficacy, is associated with the main outcome. For example, if a negative side effect is causing participants to discontinue treatment, then the results of participants remaining in the study will be biased toward a lower adverse effect profile because the participants with the adverse effects left the study. To address the possibility of such biases, many studies include measures of the rate of discontinuation due to adverse events or lack of efficacy as well as rates of the specific side effects themselves. Also, researchers typically opt to examine their results using 1 or more of 3 types of analyses: *per-protocol analysis*, *intent-to-treat* (*ITT*) *analysis*, and *last observation carried forward* (*LOCF*) *analysis*.

The *per-protocol analysis* will analyze only intervention participants who completed all or a minimum proportion of the protocol. For example, a per-protocol analysis may only involve participants who completed a certain number of visits or completed a certain number of doses. By excluding individuals who did not complete certain components of the intervention, evaluation of outcomes is more clearly and specifically linked to aspects of the intervention. If one includes those who did not complete the intervention, then outcomes may be affected by the deviations from protocol. Individuals completing certain aspects of the protocol may be different from those who do not complete such aspects. Such differences between those completing and not completing the protocol may contribute to differences in participant outcomes. A per-protocol analysis may present results that are not generalizable to the typical population not following the protocol. Another disadvantage of per-protocol analysis is that by excluding participants who did not complete certain parts of the protocol, the sample size declines and causes a decrease in the power of the study.

The *ITT analysis* includes all randomized participants according to their assignment regardless of their adherence to the treatment protocol.[14] In this situation, the researchers retain participants lost to follow-up to help improve sample size and power. However, researchers have to be careful to suggest that the intervention contributed to outcomes because the analysis includes participants who did not complete the intervention. ITT analysis involving various outcomes may not be possible because outcome measures may not be available without participant participation. For example, if participants do not complete an inventory, it will not be possible to include the participants in the ITT analysis. ITT analysis works well with data that can be collected independent of the participant's participation. Including all randomized participants in the analysis also avoids the problem that arises from uneven early discontinuation between study groups. Additionally, ITT analysis evaluates the potential effects of treatment policy rather than the effects of the treatment itself. This may prove useful in developing protocol for future clinical studies.

An example of ITT analysis can be found in a study by Montori and Guyatt.[13] Of 200 participants at risk for stroke, 100 were randomized to receive acetylsalicylic acid (ASA) and then surgery after a 1-month waiting period, whereas the other 100 participants were randomized to receive ASA alone.[13] During the waiting period, 10 ASA plus surgery participants experienced a stroke, the primary outcome of the study. A stroke might render them unfit to receive the surgery. The other 90 ASA plus surgery participants went on to receive surgery, and of those 90, 10 additional participants had strokes. Because randomization should evenly distribute baseline characteristics across both study groups, we should expect that the ASA-only group (no surgery) would also be destined to experience the same number of strokes in the month following the start of treatment (10 strokes) and thereafter (also 10 strokes). Thus, the ASA-only group has a primary outcome incidence of 20%. If investigators exclude the 10 participants who experienced a stroke in the month prior to surgery, then ASA plus surgery appears to have a better success rate (10/90 = 11%) than ASA alone (20/100 = 20%). This is misleading, because all 20 participants across both groups who had a stroke in the month following randomization experienced it under the same circumstances. In an ITT analysis, we see that surgery has little effect because the rate of stroke for each treatment group turns out to be 20% (20/100).[13]

LOCF analysis is similar to ITT analysis in that it maintains participants in the analysis despite their violations of study protocol and loss to follow-up. In LOCF analysis, the researcher takes the last valid data point of a given measure and uses it for future data points. For example, a participant drops out of a trial 3 months into a 9-month study. The researcher will take the participant's values at 3 months and incorporate them into the analyses at 9 months. Such an approach differs from ITT analysis because ITT does not take earlier available data and input as data for uncollected time points. ITT analysis examines only final collected data points on all study participants regardless of protocol violations. An advantage of an LOCF analysis is that, like ITT analysis, it maintains participants in the analysis and improves sample size and power. The primary disadvantage of LOCF analysis is that imputation of earlier values may reduce the impact of the intervention.

As a result of the advantages and disadvantages of these different analytic approaches, researchers will often use more than one approach in their analysis. If 2 or more analyses produce similar results, then this increases confidence in the conclusions of the trial. If the results differ using the different approaches, ITT analysis generally takes precedence because it preserves the value of randomization and can only cause results to be biased in a negative way and favor the null hypothesis.[6] In general, it is less problematic if the results underestimate a treatment's effect (type II error) than overestimate it (type I error). In the study on Web-based antidepressant monitoring, we decide to do both a per-protocol analysis and ITT analysis. The ITT analysis will be conducted on antidepressant adherence because we have access to the participant's refill records independent of their withdrawal from the study. The per-protocol analysis will analyze all participants who used the web-based self-management tool at least once a month during the study period.

When evaluating a study, researchers should reflect on the study's *internal and external validity*. Internal validity of a study examines the extent to which the research design has eliminated as many extraneous factors as possible that might contribute to the relationship being explored. A study with high internal validity allows the researcher to make a stronger statement that Variable A is related to or can cause Effect A. Conversely, a study with low internal validity would be hard to interpret because there would be many factors other than Variable A that might have contributed to Effect A. External validity relates to the extent to which the study can be applied to others in the population who might benefit from the intervention. External validity is another term that refers to the generalizability of the study, a concept introduced earlier in the chapter. It is important to assess how a study using controlled conditions can be applied to the real-world setting and to other members of the population not represented by the study sample. The more a study sample and procedures reflect the actual population and typical day-to-day procedures, the more likely study results can be applied to the larger nonstudy population.

■ Clinical and Statistical Significance

Another important point to consider when evaluating results is the distinction between clinical and statistical significance. A result can be statistically significant but not clinically significant. It is always important in clinical trials to evaluate the extent to which results are clinically meaningful. For example, a study finds that a drug significantly lowers blood pressure by 5 mm Hg. However, a physician asks herself if 5 mm Hg will make a significant clinical impact on the participant's risk for a heart attack. All researchers need to consider this important distinction when interpreting study findings.

■ Summary

In this chapter, we have reviewed the key components of developing, implementing, and evaluating an RCT. TABLES 6-2, 6-3, and 6-4 provide concise summaries/checklists of all the key considerations related to RCT development, implementation, and evaluation identified in this chapter. Although such trials are expensive and time consuming to carry out, most researchers would agree they are considered one of the strongest research designs to test and answer important clinical questions. More RCTs are being conducted given national scientific interest in comparative effectiveness research showing

Table 6-2	Development of an RCT

✓ Selection of study participants
- ○ Determine number of comparison groups.
  - • 1 vs 2 or 1 vs 2 vs 3
  - • Intervention group (treatment) vs control group (standard care/placebo)
- ○ Determine type of study design.
  - • Parallel
  - • Crossover
- ○ Establish inclusion and exclusion criteria.
- ○ Maintain generalizability of study population.

✓ Determination of sample size
- ○ Determine type of statistical analysis being used.
- ○ Set probabilities.
  - • Type I error (α error)
  - • Type II error (β error)
- ○ Calculate desired effect size.
- ○ Calculate power.
- ○ Anticipate attrition.

✓ Recruitment of study participants
- ○ Promote trial through creative announcements.
- ○ Offer financial incentives.
- ○ Describe benefits.

✓ Assignment of study participants
- ○ Avoid selection and ascertainment biases.
- ○ Allow randomization.
  - • Block randomization
  - • Stratified block randomization (restricted randomization)
- ○ Consider blinding.
  - • Single blinding (participant only)
  - • Double blinded (participant and investigator)

✓ Consent and ethical considerations
- ○ Obtain informed consent.
- ○ Obtain ethical review by institutional review board.
- ○ Evaluate safety and effectiveness through data and safety monitoring board.

Table 6-3	Implementation of an RCT

✓ Assess program fidelity.
  ○ Systematic and consistent implementation of intervention
  ○ Concise description of the length of intervention
  ○ Determine when outcomes will be collected
✓ Maximize adherence to study protocol and minimize dropout.
✓ Ensure follow-up monitoring plans.
✓ Consider prestudy phase (screening before randomization).
✓ Consider run-in period to test for adherence.
✓ Data collection should avoid bias.
  ○ Hawthorne effect
  ○ Surveillance bias
  ○ Interviewer bias
  ○ Social desirability bias
  ○ Recall bias

how one approach is significantly better than another approach. Meta-analyses and systematic reviews will often restrict their sample to only RCTs. Through RCTs, we strengthen the quality of evidence for which clinicians and researchers can develop best medical practices and guidelines that can significantly impact participant outcomes.

Table 6-4	Evaluation of an RCT

✓ Consider lack of valid data due to participant withdrawal.
  ○ Adverse events
  ○ Developed conditions that make them unable to remain in study
  ○ Enrollment in another trial
  ○ Moved away
  ○ Death
✓ Interpret results based on data due to loss of follow-up.
  ○ Per-protocol
  ○ Intent-to-treat (ITT)
  ○ Last observation carried forward (LOCF)
✓ Evaluate internal and external validity of results.
✓ Determine distinction between clinical and statistical significance.

■ References

1. Rossouw JE, Anderson GL, Prentice RL, et al. Risks and benefits of estrogen plus progestin in healthy postmenopausal women: principal results from the Women's Health Initiative randomized controlled trial. *JAMA*. 2002;288:321–333.

2. Anderson GL, Limacher M, Assaf AR, et al. Effects of conjugated equine estrogen in postmenopausal women with hysterectomy: the Women's Health Initiative randomized controlled trial. *JAMA*. 2004;291:1701–1712.

3. Sridharan L, Greenland P. Editorial policies and publication bias. *Arch Intern Med*. 2009;169:1022–1023.

4. Walsh BT, Seidman SN, Sysko R, et al. Placebo response in studies of major depression: variable, substantial, and growing. *JAMA*. 2002;287:1840–1847.

5. Rief W, Nestoriuc Y, Weiss S, et al. Meta-analysis of the placebo response in antidepressant trials. *J Affect Disord*. 2009;118:1–8.

6. Cummings SR, Grady D, Hulley SB. *Designing an Experiment: Clinical Trials I, II. Designing Clinical Research*. 3rd ed. Philadelphia, PA: Lippincott Williams & Wilkins; 2007.

7. Chin RY, Lee BY. *Principles and Practice of Clinical Trial Medicine*. Boston, MA: Academic; 2008.

8. Cohen J. *Statistical Power Analysis for the Behavioral Sciences*. 2nd ed. Hillsdale, NJ: Lawrence Erlbaum Associates; 1988.

9. Emanuel EJ, Grady C, Couch RA, et al, eds. *Oxford Textbook of Clinical Research Ethics*. Oxford, United Kingdom: Oxford University Press; 2008.

10. Buerki RA, Vottero LD. *Ethical Responsibility in Pharmacy Practice*. 2nd ed. Madison, WI: American Institute of the History of Pharmacy; 2002.

11. Reverby SM, ed. *Tuskegee's Truths: Rethinking the Tuskegee Syphilis Study (Studies in Social Medicine)*. Chapel Hill, NC University of North Carolina Press; 2000.

12. Molinder HK. The development of cimetidine: 1964–1976. A human story. *J Clin Gastroenterol*. 1994;19:248–254.

13. Montori VM, Guyatt GH. Intention-to-treat principle. *CMAJ*. 2001;165:1339–1341.

14. LaValley MP. Intent-to-treat analysis of randomized clinical trials. ACR/ARHP Annual Scientific Meeting Orlando. October 27, 2003. http://people.bu.edu/mlava/ ITT%20Workshop.pdf. Accessed July 2009.

Systematic Reviews and Meta-Analyses

Gerald E. Schumacher, PhD

Learning Objectives

- Distinguish between a systematic review and meta-analysis.
- Explain the utility of systematic reviews and meta-analyses in clinical practice.
- Identify the key characteristics of a good systematic review.
- Describe the key steps to conducting a systematic review.
- Explain the key statistics in performing meta-analyses.
- Analyze a meta-analysis for appropriateness and biases.
- Describe the strengths and weaknesses of systematic reviews and meta-analyses.

■ Introduction

When a single investigator or a group of investigators conducts an original, primary study, all of the elements of the study are transparent and in the control of the researchers. Objectives and hypotheses are stated, methodology is detailed, statistical tests are selected, and data are analyzed according to the study protocol. Even when the study is a multicenter endeavor, a single set of procedures governs the research. All investigators are expected to understand what transpires. But not every detail, rationale, or nuance of the study is reported in the published report of the work.

Herein lies the challenge and the difficulty of taking data from a study and combining them with data from other reports to aggregate data. The uninformed reader of the study is limited to discerning the result and implications as well as accessing what is printed. But combining similar studies, perhaps to increase the apparent sample size or resolve conflicts between results of studies, likely involves some differences in procedures, patient characteristics, sites, and other variables that may confound the interpretation of the aggregated data.

Thus, the researcher who seeks to find new information by combining studies recognizes that it is necessary to invoke a new set of procedures, statistical maneuvers, and evaluative limitations to facilitate moving from being the investigator who conceived an original study to becoming the investigator who extracts and aggregates what is available in publication from various studies.

■ Comparing Narrative Review, Systematic Review, and Meta-Analysis

We have all read reviews of various kinds in health care and other areas. Sometimes the review, perhaps about a drug or a disease, cites a number of articles that may have been chosen by the author to reinforce the viewpoint of the review. Often it is not clear from the report what strategy was used to select the cited articles that were selected, how many studies were not selected, why those studies were rejected, how selective the author of the review was in extracting information for inclusion while rejecting material not included, and whether the selection of the included articles leads to a bias in interpretation and conclusion of the review. What this describes is the general form of the **narrative review**, which is the least sophisticated and useful of summary reports.

In contrast, a **systematic review (SR)** is an overview and summary of primary studies that contains a statement of objectives and methods and has been conducted according to an explicit and reproducible methodology that encourages transparency.[1] SRs are essential tools for aggregating evidence and presenting the material accurately and without bias. It is estimated that more than 2500 English-language SRs are published annually.[2] These vary in rigor, sophistication, and quality.

The Cochrane Collaboration (www.cochrane.org) is the most notable purveyor of SRs.[3,4] Within the Collaboration, the Cochrane Library (www.cochrane.org/reviews/clibintro.htm) contains over 4000 reviews documenting the evidence for and against the effectiveness and appropriateness of treatments (eg, medications, surgery, education) in specific circumstances. An example of a complete Cochrane review is available online (www.cochrane.org/reviews/exreview.htm).

As summarized in TABLE 7-1, there are 7 general steps in an SR.

- *Step 1.* State precisely the objective(s) of the review and outline eligibility criteria for including or rejecting published studies for the review. This makes a clear statement to the reader of intent and the scope of the review. Eligibility criteria vary with the subject of the review but generally include items such as participants (eg, age, sex, study setting, disease/condition, and other pertinent characteristics), interventions or exposures under consideration, comparator group intervention, outcomes of the intervention being assessed, and study design.
- *Step 2.* Conduct a thorough search of the literature for primary studies that appear to meet the eligibility criteria for inclusion in the review. The most inclusive of SRs also includes unpublished reports where available and access to the

Table 7-1	General Steps in the Development of a Systematic Review

1. State objectives of the review and outline eligibility criteria for studies to be included.
2. Search the literature for studies that appear to meet the eligibility criteria.
3. Tabulate the characteristics of each trial identified and assess its methodologic quality.
4. Apply eligibility criteria and justify any exclusions.
5. For quantitative reviews, assemble and aggregate the most comprehensive data set feasible.
6. Analyze the results of the eligible studies by using statistical synthesis of data (the meta-analysis step).
7. Prepare a structured report of the review, stating objectives, methods, critical analysis of data, limitations of the review and analysis, and recommendations for use of the review.

Source: Adapted from Greenhalgh T. *How to Read a Paper: The Basics of Evidence-Based Medicine.* London, UK: BMJ Publishing Group; 1997.

original data from the published and unpublished studies. In this chapter, we restrict the SR to the much more common situation in which published articles are the only source of material for the review.

- *Step 3.* Tabulate the characteristics of each study that has the potential for inclusion as described in Step 1. After tabulation is complete, each study is evaluated for general soundness of methodology. Inadequate methodology should disqualify a study at this step.
- *Step 4.* Apply the eligibility criteria to each of the proposed studies for inclusion. Studies excluded at this step should be justified and recorded.
- *Step 5.* For quantitative reviews, assemble and then aggregate the most germane and comprehensive data set from the studies approved for inclusion in the review.
- *Step 6.* For quantitative reviews, perform the statistical assessment and synthesis of the data. This is the meta-analysis step in the procedure (meta-analysis as a technique is included when indicated as part of the overall SR process).
- *Step 7.* Prepare a structured report of the review. It should contain objectives, methods, critical analysis of data, limitations of the review and analysis, and recommendations for use of the report.

At its simplest, **meta-analysis (MA)** is a statistical synthesis of the numerical results of several trials that all examined the same question.[1] It is the quantitative component of an SR that combines the results of relevant studies to produce and investigate an estimate of the overall effect of interest. Just as all SRs do not include an MA, an MA may be conducted without using the full structure of an SR. However, it is not uncommon for authors to refer to SRs and MAs interchangeably. In this chapter, we use the more accepted approach of applying the term SR to refer to the entire process of collecting, reviewing, and reporting the evidence pertinent to a subject. MA, as noted earlier, refers just to the statistical procedure of extracting, aggregating, and analyzing data to yield a summary result; it is one of the steps in the process of preparing an SR.[3,4]

As an overview of the procedure, an MA uses appropriate aggregation and statistical techniques to calculate for each component study the "point estimate" and its associated variation for each outcome of interest followed by then calculating the resulting overall summary of data for each of the outcomes. By combining like studies to increase sample size, MA has the potential to achieve the following 5 objectives: (1) calculate an overall summary estimate of effect size of the intervention (the incremental difference between test and control interventions) with greater power and a smaller confidence interval than is achieved for any of the individual component studies; (2) resolve differences in component study conclusions by aggregating a combined, summary study; (3) explore the reasons for differences in effects between and among studies; (4) identify heterogeneity (true rather than chance variation among the outcome[s] of interest in the component individual studies) in the effects of the intervention, or differences in risk, in different subgroups; and (5) assist in achieving consensus on guidelines for treatments, procedures, conditions, and so on.[5]

Examples of Systematic Reviews and Meta-Analyses in Drug Treatment

With so many health care SRs and MAs published in English annually, it is an overwhelming task to summarize the field in a single chapter. Using a search engine and the keywords "systematic review" and "meta-analysis" yields a trove of publications to demonstrate the breadth of the applications. Also, a perusal of the Cochrane Library provides many reviews. A few recent examples from the literature involving drug therapy of widely varying conditions will be noted in this chapter.[6-10] They provide a glimpse of the spectrum of application of these analytical techniques. Then, one review will be examined in detail in this chapter.[11]

Example A

The report titled, "Systematic Review and Meta-Analysis of Evidence for Increasing Numbers of Drugs in Antiretroviral Combination Therapy," concluded that the evidence from randomized controlled trials (RCTs) supports the use of triple-drug therapy in treating human immunodeficiency virus infections.[6] Using the odds ratio for measure of relative effect, the authors conducted an SR and MA of aggregated studies of RCTs to demonstrate, first, the greater effectiveness of double-drug as opposed to single-drug therapy and, second, the even greater effectiveness of triple-drug as opposed to double-drug treatment.

Example B

In the report titled, "Prenatal Multivitamin Supplementation and Rates of Pediatric Cancers: A Meta-Analysis," investigators studied published RCTs to assess the protective effect of prenatal multivitamins on several types of pediatric cancers.[7] Using the odds ratio as a measure of risk, a protective effect of maternal ingestion of prenatal multi-vitamins was demonstrated for pediatric brain tumors, neuroblastoma, and leukemia.

Example C

In the report titled, "Meta-Analysis: Effects of Adding Salmeterol to Inhaled Corticosteroids on Serious Asthma-Related Events," researchers aggregated RCTs to study whether the incidence of severe asthma-related events differs in persons receiving salmeterol plus inhaled corticosteroids compared with inhaled corticosteroids alone.[8] They showed a decreased risk in the events when adding the corticosteroid for severe exacerbations but no change in risk for asthma-related hospitalizations or death.

Example D

The report titled, "The APPLe Study: A Randomized, Community-Based, Placebo-Controlled Trial of Azithromycin for the Prevention of Preterm Birth, with Meta-Analysis," examined an aggregation of RCTs to determine the effect of routine prophylaxis on preterm birth in high-risk populations.[9] The investigators resolved an issue by showing that there were no significant differences in outcome, using the odds ratio, between the azithromycin and placebo groups with respect to the risk of preterm birth.

Example E

In the report titled, "Treatment of Fibromyalgia Syndrome with Antidepressants: A Meta-Analysis," investigators studied the efficacy of antidepressants in the treatment of fibromyalgia syndrome by performing an MA of clinical RCTs.[10] Tricyclic and tetracyclic antidepressants (TCAs), selective serotonin reuptake inhibitors (SSRIs), serotonin and noradrenaline reuptake inhibitors (SNRIs), and monoamine oxidase inhibitors (MAOIs) were analyzed. There was very good evidence for an association of antidepressants with reduction in pain, depressed mood, and sleep disturbances. Effect sizes for pain reduction were greatest for TCAs, and smallest for SSRIs and SNRIs, with MAOIs in between.

This small sampling of recent SRs and MAs demonstrates the impact of these summative techniques on updating issues or expanding our understanding of the effects of drug treatment. Of course, an MA is only as valid as the studies included. Conclusions may change as more data become available. The Cochrane Collaboration updates their SAs as more studies are published.

■ Steps in Conducting and Interpreting Systematic Reviews and Meta-Analyses

A single chapter is inadequate to demonstrate the sophisticated techniques of SRs and MAs. Three books offer in-depth treatment of these topics.[5,12,13] The Cochrane Collaboration also offers extensive coverage of the material.[3,4] Short reviews are available in journals.[14-16]

This chapter will not focus on using the rigorous techniques for conducting these studies; instead, the emphasis is on a basic understanding, interpretation, and evaluation of published reports of SRs and MAs. A download of the prototypical article to be analyzed in this chapter is freely available in 2 forms,[11] as a full report from the *BMJ* "online first" Web site (2009;339:b2976; www.bmj.com/content/339/bmj.b2976.full) and in abridged form from the *BMJ* "print journal" (2009;339:488–493). Downloading the article will enhance interpretation of the discussion that follows.

The 7 steps in Table 7-1 will be used to review the 2009 publication, titled "Corticosteroids for Pain Relief in Sore Throat: Systematic Review and Meta-Analysis."[11] The investigators aggregated published RCTs to evaluate whether systemic corticosteroid treatment for children and adults with severe or exudative sore throat would reduce the associated pain.

Step 1: State Objectives of the Review and Outline Eligibility Criteria for Studies to Be Included

The investigators stated at the outset their intention to "evaluate whether systemic corticosteroids improve symptoms of sore throat in adults and children." Further, they hypothesized that "… corticosteroids would offer symptomatic relief from sore throat because of their anti-inflammatory effects and undertook a systematic review to examine the effect."[11]

The eligibility criteria for inclusion of articles for the SR and MA spring from the previously mentioned objectives. In the Methods section, reference is made to including only RCTs "… comparing systematic corticosteroids with placebo, in children and adults in outpatient settings." Also, studies included were of "… patients with clinical signs of acute tonsillitis or pharyngitis and patients with a clinical syndrome of 'sore throat' (painful throat, odynophagia)."[11]

The investigators meet the requirements of Step 1.

Step 2: Search the Literature for Studies That Appear to Meet the Eligibility Criteria

In the Methods section, the investigators stated that they searched "… Medline, Embase, the Cochrane Library, the Database of reviews of effectiveness (DARE) and the NHS Health Economics Database." Search terms included "upper respiratory tract infection," "pharyngitis," "tonsillitis," "sore throat," "corticosteroids," and viral and bacterial upper respiratory pathogens. They excluded studies of "infectious mononucleosis, sore throat following tonsillectomy or intubation, or peritonsillar abscess."[11]

Further detail describing article selection based on content of the abstract is provided: "Two authors independently reviewed the title and abstracts of electronic searches, obtaining the full articles to assess for relevance where necessary. Disagreements were resolved by discussion with a third author."[11]

The investigators meet the requirements of Step 2.

Step 3: Tabulate the Characteristics of Each Trial Indentified and Assess Its Methodologic Quality

As stated in the Methods section, as in Step 2, "Two authors independently assessed study quality and extracted data using an extraction template. Disagreements were documented and resolved by discussion with a third author." Methodologic quality of studies was assessed by "... allocation concealment, randomization, comparability of groups on baseline characteristics, blinding, treatment adherence, and percentage participation."[11]

The primary outcomes recorded by the authors included the proportion of participants with improvement or complete resolution of symptoms, mean times to onset of pain relief, and complete resolution of pain. Additionally, secondary outcomes were recorded as reduction of pain measured by visual analog scale, adverse reactions requiring discontinuation of treatment, rates of relapse, and days missed from school or work.

The investigators meet the requirements of Step 3.

Step 4: Apply Eligibility Criteria and Justify Any Exclusions

The investigators give a flowchart of search results in Figure 1 of their online report. The flowchart is not included in the print edition manuscript. "Of the 3257 potentially relevant records identified, 26 were relevant to sore throat, tonsillitis, or pharyngitis. Of these, 17 studies were further excluded because they examined postoperative or postintubation sore throat, included inpatients, did not have a placebo group, or were duplicate publications. Of the nine that fully met our inclusion criteria, one was excluded for not describing the method of randomization."[11] Of the original cache of 3257 potentially relevant reports, 8 studies survived the inclusion criteria and were used to conduct the MA in Step 5. Characteristics of the 8 studies are reported in Table 1 of the online report.

The investigators meet the requirements of Step 4.

Step 5: For Quantitative Reviews, Assemble and Aggregate the Most Comprehensive Data Set Feasible

For the 8 qualifying studies used for analysis, Table 1 of the online report includes full inclusion characteristics of the reports. The table is not included in the print edition manuscript, but reference is made to the availability of the table in the online report. In addition, Table 2 of the online report records the characteristics supporting the methodologic quality of the 8 studies; assessed were allocation concealment, randomization, comparability of groups at baseline, blinding, percent participation, and provision of care apart from the intervention.

The investigators meet the requirements of Step 5.

Step 6: Analyze the Results of the Eligible Studies Using Statistical Synthesis of Data (the MA Step)

Each of the 8 eligible studies is individually assessed for heterogeneity. Ideally, each of the studies shares the same characteristics and methodology so that the investigator could imagine that all the studies could be combined with equal weight to achieve an overall summed value for each measure of outcome. But in reality, this does not happen, so it is necessary to determine how consistent the studies are (ie, how well the data of the studies fit with the data from the other studies). The most common approach for doing this is to assess the homogeneity of each report. To do this, the corollary heterogeneity is the trait evaluated.

Tests of heterogeneity seek to determine whether there are genuine differences underlying the results of the studies (heterogeneity) or whether the variation in findings is merely the effect of chance (homogeneity).[17] See FIGURES 7-1 and 7-2, which we will soon discuss in detail. Notice that the dots represent the point estimates, and the length of the horizontal lines embracing each of the dots represents the percent confidence interval (usually 95%) for the point estimate. The most casual assessment of the extent of heterogeneity comes from inspecting whether each of the confidence intervals overlaps to some extent the intervals for the other studies. Studies that do not overlap each other will likely turn out on more sophisticated analysis to be heterogeneous with the other studies. The greater the extent of heterogeneity among the studies, the less likely it is that the overall summary result of the aggregated studies will be an accurate reflection of the true value.

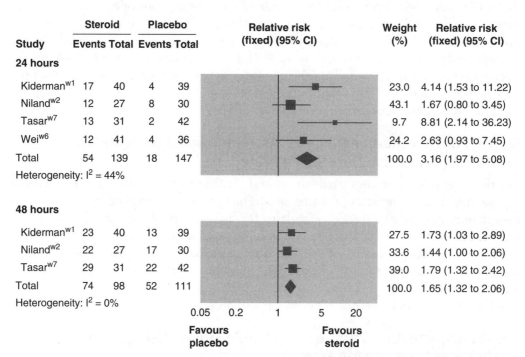

FIGURE 7-1 Effect of corticosteroids on number of patients experiencing complete pain relief at 24 and 48 hours. CI, confidence interval.

Source: Reprinted with permission from Hayward G, Thompson M, Heneghan C, et al. Corticosteroids for pain relief in sore throat: systematic review and meta-analysis. *BMJ.* 2009;339:488–493 (online: 2009;339:b2976).

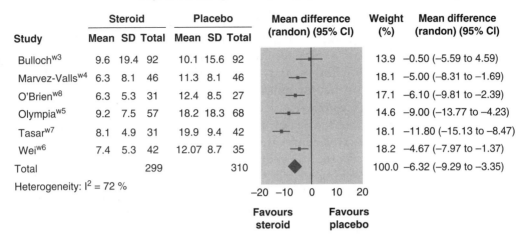

Study	Steroid			Placebo			Mean difference (randon) (95% CI)	Weight (%)	Mean difference (randon) (95% CI)
	Mean	SD	Total	Mean	SD	Total			
Bulloch[w3]	9.6	19.4	92	10.1	15.6	92		13.9	−0.50 (−5.59 to 4.59)
Marvez-Valls[w4]	6.3	8.1	46	11.3	8.1	46		18.1	−5.00 (−8.31 to −1.69)
O'Brien[w8]	6.3	5.3	31	12.4	8.5	27		17.1	−6.10 (−9.81 to −2.39)
Olympia[w5]	9.2	7.5	57	18.2	18.3	68		14.6	−9.00 (−13.77 to −4.23)
Tasar[w7]	8.1	4.9	31	19.9	9.4	42		18.1	−11.80 (−15.13 to −8.47)
Wei[w6]	7.4	5.3	42	12.07	8.7	35		18.2	−4.67 (−7.97 to −1.37)
Total			299			310		100.0	−6.32 (−9.29 to −3.35)

Heterogeneity: $I^2 = 72\%$

Favours steroid   Favours placebo

FIGURE 7-2 Effect of corticosteroids on mean time to onset of pain relief in hours. CI, confidence interval; SD, standard deviation.

Source: Reprinted with permission from Hayward G, Thompson M, Heneghan C, et al. Corticosteroids for pain relief in sore throat: systematic review and meta-analysis. *BMJ.* 2009;339:488–493 (online: 2009;339:b2976).

Two commonly reported quantitative tests of heterogeneity and associated inconsistency among studies are the I^2 index and the Q statistic resulting from Cochran's χ^2 test for homogeneity. The former test is considered the more reliable of the 2 tests.[17] I^2 denotes the percentage of the total variation across the included studies that is due to heterogeneity; the value of the statistic ranges from 0% to 100%, with 0% reflecting no heterogeneity (complete homogeneity). Although there is no consensus on what threshold of I^2 separates homogeneity from heterogeneity, values above 50% caution wariness in interpretation of the results. In these situations, calculating an overall summary effect for the MA is likely not useful. Subgroup analysis of the studies may then be used to reveal the source of the inconsistencies.

Two different statistical approaches to assessing the summary outcomes of an MA are used depending on the extent of heterogeneity for the component studies. When heterogeneity is modest to low (perhaps $I^2 < 50\%$), a fixed-effects model of analysis is used.[5,18] With this approach, the interpretation is based on the studies actually included in the MA. The assumption is that the treatment effect is the same in each of the included studies and any observed variation (which leads to some numerical measure of heterogeneity) is due to sampling error or chance alone. When heterogeneity is high (perhaps $I^2 > 50\%$), a random-effects model is used, also known as the DerSimonian and Laird method.[5,19] In this case, the interpretation assumes that the results observed from the studies used in the MA reflect a random sample of some hypothetical population of studies. Therefore the assumption is that the studies included yield an aggregated mean treatment effect, but that each of the component studies produces a mean effect that varies about the summary result. Figures 7-1 and 7-2 show the use of fixed-effects and random-effects models, respectively.

Heterogeneity can be clinically or statistically based.[5,20] Clinical heterogeneity is qualitative in nature and results when characteristics or design of the intervention (eg, subjects, age, severity, dose, treatment duration, effects of the intervention on different subgroups) may be responsible for the variation in outcomes observed. Statistical heterogeneity is quantitative in nature, resulting from significant variation in values for the outcome measures among studies, and urges a subsequent examination of clinical heterogeneity to explain how it contributes to the variation in results observed.

Outcomes are commonly assessed with continuous (using means) or dichotomous (using risk ratio or odds ratio) scales of measure. Whichever measure is used, the contribution of each study to the aggregated database is weighted by some variable. Usually this weighting reflects the variability of the study data about the point estimate.[5] One measure of estimating weight is by the reciprocal of the measure used for study variability. To think of this visually, the wider the confidence interval is about the point estimate (a measure of data variability in a study), the less the study contributes (is weighted) in the overall aggregation and summary result. In general, studies with a large sample size have a greater impact on aggregated results than smaller studies. Differing scales of measure and weighting are reflected in Figures 7-1 and 7-2.

Calculating the results for an MA is usually done using specialized MA software. Two common examples are RevMan (www.cc-ims.net/revman), the software used by the Cochrane Collaborative, and Comprehensive Meta-Analysis (www.meta-analysis.com).

Figures 7-1 and 7-2, which come from the example study we are discussing,[11] represent the most common method for displaying individual and aggregate study data for an MA. The presentation, referred to as a forest plot,[21] graphs the outcome data measure on the horizontal axis and each of the individual component studies, usually in chronological order, on the vertical axis. The vertical line that runs through the various study results is the line of "no treatment effect." When the outcome data are continuous (mean difference), the value is 0. When the data are dichotomous (risk ratio, odds ratio), the value is 1. The point estimate for each study is denoted with a box, and its size is proportional to the weighted contribution of the study. The line that includes the point estimate is the confidence interval for the individual result. The overall summary result is usually depicted with a diamond spanning the width of the confidence interval. If the diamond does not cross the line of no treatment effect, the summary result is statistically significant at the level of confidence (typically 95%) used in the analysis.

Recall that in Step 5, of the original cache of 3257 potentially relevant reports, 8 studies survived the inclusion criteria and were used to conduct the MA. This resulted in an aggregated sample of 743 patient records (roughly equally divided between adults and children), with patients divided somewhat equally between exudative sore throat and positive laboratory report for group A β-hemolytic *Streptococcus*. Patient records were obtained from emergency departments and general practice settings in 4 countries, choosing among betamethasone, dexamethasone, and prednisone as the corticosteroids used. All 8 studies prescribed antibiotics and permitted simple analgesia to both treatment and placebo groups. As noted earlier in Step 4, characteristics of the 8 studies are reported in Table 1 of the online report.

Figure 7-1 is the same as Figures 2 and 1 in the online and print versions, respectively, of example article.[11] Referring to Figure 7-1, the data reported complete resolution of pain at 24 and 48 hours for the 4 and 3 studies included, respectively. A fixed-effects model, as indicated in the figure, was used because the heterogeneity index, I^2, was modest (< 50%). The weighting of the studies was recorded showing that the highest contributor in the 24-hour study was weighted nearly 5 times that of the lowest contributor. This is confirmed visually by the comparative width of the confidence intervals for 2 studies. For the 48-hour study, there was no heterogeneity ($I^2 = 0\%$), and the relative width of the confidence intervals was predictive of the more similar weighting of studies than in the 24-hour study. In this particular configuration of the relative risk measure, a ratio greater than 1 showed the ameliorative benefit of using corticosteroids, and a ratio less than 1 denoted the lack of a corticosteroid effect. At 24 hours, the overall summary result was that patients using corticosteroids were 3.16 times as likely to have complete resolution of pain as patients in the no corticosteroid group; at 48 hours, the intervention cohort was 1.65 times as likely to benefit as the placebo group. The values are statistically significant ($P < 0.001$). This is also displayed by the overall summary confidence intervals for the 24- and 48-hour studies that did not cross the vertical line of no treatment effect (1 for a dichotomous measure of outcome).

In Figure 7-2 (Figures 3 and 2 in the online and print versions of the study,[11] respectively), the data show the outcome of mean time to onset of pain relief in hours, recorded as the mean difference between intervention and placebo. For the 6 studies included, there was worrisome heterogeneity ($I^2 = 72\%$) as reinforced by noting that some of the confidence intervals for the studies did not overlap. This was attributed to the wide variation in response times for the patients. When heterogeneity is high, the random-effects statistical model is used as indicated in the figure. Despite this, the results showed that corticosteroid users on average received onset of pain relief some 6 hours earlier (95% confidence interval of roughly 3–9 hours) than patients not using the intervention. The overall confidence interval did not cross the vertical line of no treatment effect (0 for a continuous measure of outcome; $P < 0.001$).

There is, of course, much more data and narrative in the online and print versions of the study[11] than we have discussed here. Of note is the requisite posting of limitations in the MA, including the following: (1) all 8 studies provided antibiotics to the intervention and placebo patients, making it impossible to assess the independent effect of corticosteroid administration, separate from antibiotic use, on sore throat symptoms; (2) some data were not reported in the included studies; (3) one study contributed significantly more heterogeneity to the aggregated results than the other reports, leading to a welcome decrease in I^2 value when the study was omitted (the Taser trial); (4) the mean time to onset of pain outcome measure was limited by recall bias, a result of retrospective assessment and subjective recall; and (5) it was not possible to assess publication bias because there was a limited number of eligible trials.

Publication bias refers to the greater likelihood of studies reporting positive results being published than those recording negative results. This is often referred to as the "file drawer problem," eluding to the fact that some studies do not get published and thus get "filed away." This biases the distribution of effect sizes because results are generally limited to only published reports. One method of assessing the extent of this bias is through the use of a funnel plot that graphs a scatter plot of study sample sizes and corresponding effect sizes.[5,22] In general, if there is no publication bias, studies of large and small effect sizes should be distributed somewhat symmetrically around the point of overall effect size.

The investigators meet the requirements of Step 6.

Step 7: Prepare a Structured Report of the Review, Stating Objectives, Methods, Critical Analysis of Data, Limitations of the Review and Analysis, and Recommendations for Use of the Review

These 7 general steps embrace the annotated checklist of 27 items to be included when reporting an SR, shown in TABLE 7-2, as recommended in the PRISMA statement for reporting SR and MA evaluating health care interventions.[23] PRISMA is the acronym for Preferred Reporting Items for Systematic Reviews and Meta-Analyses. The statement is the consensus report of a group of 29 review authors, methodologists, clinicians, medical editors, and consumers.

The example study in its full online version meets the requirement of Step 7.

Although it does not include all of the recommended steps in the PRISMA checklist, the example study does provide more than enough narrative to fully inform the reader of the objectives, implementation, analysis, and interpretation of the SR and MA. The printed version is abridged, clearly a decision of the journal editor and not the authors, but the manuscript does refer the reader to additional details in the online version.

■ Summary

SRs and MAs make valuable contributions to the literature of assessment. Properly conducted, they have the potential to forcefully summarize the magnitude of treatment effects, when individual studies leave the question(s) unresolved. They have the potential to reveal heterogeneity in studies that may help to clear confusion in decision making. And finally, they have the potential to assist in the development of treatment guidelines.

However, Petitti appropriately summarizes some cautions[5]:

> Meta-analysis is an observational, not an experimental method. The main value of meta-analysis, even meta-analysis of individual trials, is to generate hypotheses, not to test them. All meta-analysis is essentially exploratory analysis.
>
>   Meta-analysis can help set the stage for large trials. It may be a guide to clinical decision-making until large trials can be completed. It is not a substitute for conduct of large trials and should not be used as such.[5]

Table 7-2		Checklist of Items to Include When Reporting a Systematic Review or Meta-Analysis
Section/Topic	#	Checklist Item

Title

| Title | 1 | Identify the report as a systematic review, meta-analysis, or both. |

Abstract

| Structured summary | 2 | Provide a structured summary, including, as applicable: background; objectives; data sources; study eligibility criteria, participants, and interventions; study appraisal and synthesis methods; results; limitations; conclusions and implications of key findings; and systematic review registration number. |

Introduction

| Rationale | 3 | Describe the rationale for the review in the context of what is already known. |
| Objectives | 4 | Provide an explicit statement of questions being addressed with reference to participants, interventions, comparisons, outcomes, and study design (PICOS). |

Methods

Protocol and registration	5	Indicate if a review protocol exists and if and where it can be accessed (eg, Web address), and, if available, provide registration information including registration number.
Eligibility criteria	6	Specify study characteristics (eg, PICOS, length of follow-up) and report characteristics (eg, years considered, language, publication status) used as criteria for eligibility, giving rationale.
Information sources	7	Describe all information sources (eg, databases with dates of coverage, contact with study authors to identify additional studies) in the search and date last searched.
Search	8	Present full electronic search strategy for at least one database, including any limits used, such that it could be repeated.
Study selection	9	State the process for selecting studies (ie, screening, eligibility) included in the systematic review and, if applicable, included in the meta-analysis.
Data collection process	10	Describe method of data extraction from reports (eg, piloted forms, independently, in duplicate) and any processes for obtaining and confirming data from investigators.
Data items	11	List and define all variables for which data were sought (eg, PICOS, funding sources) and any assumptions and simplifications made.
Risk of bias in individual studies	12	Describe methods used for assessing risk of bias of individual studies (including specification of whether this was done at the study or outcome level) and how this information is to be used in any data synthesis.
Summary measures	13	State the principal summary measures (eg, risk ratio, difference in means).

(continues)

Table 7-2		Checklist of Items to Include When Reporting a Systematic Review or Meta-Analysis (Continued)
Section/Topic	#	Checklist Item
Synthesis of results	14	Describe the methods of handling data and combining results of studies, if done, including measures of consistency (eg, I^2) for each meta-analysis.
Risk of bias across studies	15	Specify any assessment of risk of bias that may affect the cumulative evidence (eg, publication bias, selective reporting within studies).
Additional analyses	16	Describe methods of additional analyses (eg, sensitivity or subgroup analyses, meta-regression), if done, indicating which were prespecified.
Results		
Study selection	17	Give numbers of studies screened, assessed for eligibility, and included in the review, with reasons for exclusions at each stage, ideally with a flow diagram.
Study characteristics	18	For each study, present characteristics for which data were extracted (eg, study size, PICOS, follow-up period) and provide the citations.
Risk of bias within studies	19	Present data on risk of bias of each study and, if available, any outcome-level assessment (see Item 12).
Results of individual studies	20	For all outcomes considered (benefits or harms), present, for each tudy: (a) simple summary data for each intervention group and (b) effect estimates and confidence intervals, ideally with a forest plot.
Synthesis of results	21	Present results of each meta-analysis done, including confidence intervals and measures of consistency.
Risk of bias across studies	22	Present results of any assessment of risk of bias across studies (see Item 15).
Additional analysis	23	Give results of additional analyses, if done (eg, sensitivity or subgroup analyses, meta-regression [see Item 16]).
Discussion		
Summary of evidence	24	Summarize the main findings including the strength of evidence for each main outcome; consider their relevance to key groups (eg, health care providers, users, and policy makers).
Limitations	25	Discuss limitations at study and outcome level (eg, risk of bias) and at review level (eg, incomplete retrieval of identified research, reporting bias).
Conclusions	26	Provide a general interpretation of the results in the context of other evidence and implications for future research.
Funding		
Funding	27	Describe sources of funding for the systematic review and other support (eg, supply of data), and role of funders for the systematic review.

Source: Adapted from Liberati A, Altman D, Tetzlaff J, et al. The PRISMA statement for reporting systematic reviews and meta-analysis of studies that evaluate health are interventions: explanation and elaboration. *PLoS Med.* 2009;6:1–28.

■ References

1. Greenhalgh T. *How to Read a Paper: The Basics of Evidence-Based Medicine*. London, United Kingdom: BMJ Publishing Group; 1997.

2. Moher D, Tetzlaff J, Tricco A, et al. Epidemiology and reporting characteristics of systematic reviews. *PLoS Med*. 2007;4:e78.

3. Higgins J, Green S, eds. *Cochrane Handbook for Systematic Reviews of Interventions*. Version 5.0.2. http://www.cochrane-handbook.org. Accessed January 21, 1010.

4. Cochrane Collaboration. The Cochrane Collaboration open learning material. Systematic reviews and meta-analyses. 2002. http://www.cochrane-net.org/openlearning/HTML/mod3-2.htm. Accessed November 12, 2009.

5. Petitti D. *Meta-Analysis, Decision Analysis, and Cost-Effectiveness Analysis*. 2nd ed. New York, NY: Oxford University Press; 2000.

6. Jordan R, Gold L, Cummins C, et al. Systematic review and meta-analysis of evidence for increasing numbers of drugs in antiretroviral combination therapy. *BMJ*. 2002;324:757–760.

7. Goh Y, Bollano E, Einaraon T, et al. Prenatal multivitamin supplementation and rates of pediatric cancers: a meta-analysis. *Clin Pharmacol Ther*. 2007;81:685–691.

8. Bateman E, Nelson H, Bousquet J, et al. Meta-analysis: effects of adding salmeterol to inhaled corticosteroids on serious asthma-related events. *Arch Intern Med*. 2008;149:33–42.

9. van den Broek N, White A, Goodall M, et al. The APPLe study: a randomized, community-based placebo-controlled trial of azithromycin for the prevention of preterm birth, with meta-analysis. *PLoS Med*. 2009;6:1–8.

10. Häuser W, Bernardy K, Üçeyler N, et al. Treatment of fibromyalgia syndrome with antidepressants: a meta-analysis. *JAMA*. 2009;301:198–209.

11. Hayward G, Thompson M, Heneghan C, et al. Corticosteroids for pain relief in sore throat: systematic review and meta-analysis. *BMJ*. 2009;339:488–493 (online: 2009;339:b2976).

12. Egger M, Smith G, Altman D, eds. *Systematic Reviews in Health Care*. London, United Kingdom: BMJ Books; 2001.

13. Hedges L, Higgins J, Rothstein H. *Introduction to Meta-Analysis*. West Sussex, United Kingdom: John Wiley & Sons; 2009.

14. Pai M, McCulloch M, Gorman J, et al. Systematic reviews and meta-analyses: an illustrated, step-by-step guide. *Natl Med J India*. 2004;17:86–95.

15. Green S. Systematic reviews and meta-analysis. *Singapore Med J*. 2005;46:270–274.

16. Akobeng A. Understanding systematic reviews and meta-analysis. *Arch Dis Child*. 2005;90:845–848.

17. Higgins J, Thompson S, Deeks J, et al. Measuring inconsistency in meta-analyses. *BMJ*. 2003;327:557–560.

18. Mantel N, Haenszel W. Statistical aspects of the analysis of data from retrospective studies of disease. *J Natl Cancer Inst*. 1959;22:719–748.

19. DerSimonian R, Laird N. Meta-analysis in clinical trials. *Control Clin Trials*. 1986;7:177–188.

20. Thompson S. Why sources of heterogeneity in meta-analysis should be investigated. *BMJ*. 1994;309:1351–1355.

21. Lewis S, Clarke M. Forest plots: trying to see the wood and the trees. *BMJ*. 2001;322:1479–1480.

22. Sterne J, Egger M. Funnel plots for detecting bias in meta-analysis: guidelines on choice of axis. *J Clin Epidemiol*. 2001;54:1045–1046.

23. Liberati A, Altman D, Tetzlaff J, et al. The PRISMA statement for reporting systematic reviews and meta-analysis of studies that evaluate health are interventions: explanation and elaboration. *PLoS Med*. 2009;6:1–28.

Medical and Prescription Claims Databases

Donald G. Klepser, PhD, MBA

Learning Objectives

- Construct a valid argument for using medical and prescription claims databases in health outcomes research.

- Understand the primary purpose of medical and prescription claims databases and how that affects their use in research.

- Describe common types of studies conducted using medical and prescription claims data.

- Identify the key information contained in a claims database.

- Differentiate between inpatient, outpatient, and prescription databases.

- Discuss the advantages and disadvantages of using claims databases for conducting outcomes research.

- Discuss the challenges associated with determining actual care from claims data.

- Describe processes by which researchers can control for confounding in claims-based research.

■ Introduction

In a perfect world, researchers would be able to answer all questions definitively using only the best possible methodologies. In health outcomes research, that would mean conducting all research using randomized controlled trials (RCTs), which are the accepted "gold standard" for determining cause and effect. Unfortunately, we do not live in a perfect world and things like ethical considerations, patient safety, and costs (both to the patient and to the researcher) influence research methodology and the questions that can be answered. Therefore, we have to look at other methods for answering questions where it would be either unethical or cost prohibitive to conduct an RCT.

One method is to conduct research using existing data. These data may come from surveys, disease registries, medical charts, electronic health records, or administrative databases. Technologic innovations have made these data more widely available to researchers than at any time in the past. Although all of these secondary data sources can be useful in conducting research, this chapter will focus on medical and prescription claims databases as they exist in the United States, which vary in number compared with nations that have socialized health care systems including reimbursement (eg, Canada, United Kingdom).

Medical and prescription claims databases were not developed as research tools. Rather, they are a byproduct of the need for an efficient system to conduct financial transactions within the health care system. Because they are not present at the time of service, third-party payers need to know (1) who provided what services, (2) for whom the services were provided, (3) when the services were provided, (4) for what conditions, and (5) at what charge. With this information, they can determine if and how much they should reimburse the providers of services.

Information within the claims databases can also be used by insurers for other internal clinical and business purposes such as utilization reviews and underwriting. The use of claims databases in research is a relatively recent occurrence. In addition to the recognition of valuable information contained in the databases (eg, real-world utilization patterns), the use of claims data for research purposes has been made possible by recent advances in computing power that makes it possible for researchers to handle large data sets.

After a brief description of medical and prescription claims databases, this chapter will discuss the advantages and disadvantages of using the data and the types of studies conducted using the data. The remainder of the chapter will provide practical information on sources of claims data and how to conduct a study using claims data. Throughout the chapter, we will use a case to illustrate a study conducted using claims databases.

■ What Exactly Is a Claims Database?

Generally speaking, claims data consist of a variety (enrollment, medical, and prescription) of databases (TABLE 8-1). Linking these databases allows the researcher to get a clear sense of the care delivered and patients' utilization. Prospective researchers should be aware that they may not have access to all of these databases depending on the source of their data. Arguably in the United States, one centralized database of all health care services provided to patients, including medical, diagnostics, and prescriptions is the database of the Veterans Administration.

Many employers contract separately for their prescription benefit. This means that a researcher getting data from the primary health insurer may not have access to the prescription claims database. Likewise, a researcher getting data from a pharmacy benefits manager (PBM) is unlikely to have access to medical claims. Although a significant amount of health care research is conducted annually, without access to the population's entire claims history, there are definite limitations to the research that can

Table 8-1	Claims Database Files		
File Type	Description	Unit of Observation	Common Variables
Enrollment file	The insurer's record of who has coverage at any given time	Member level	• Unique member identifier • Dates of coverage • Date of birth • Sex • County of residence • Plan design variables
Medical claims			

Institutional/ hospital claims	Care provided by inpatient and outpatient institutions, including all hospital stays	Episode level	• Unique member identifier
			• Unique encounter identifier
			• Admission and discharge dates
			• Diagnoses
			• Procedures
			• Costs
			  ○ Total
			  ○ Patient
			  ○ Insurer/employer

Provider/ physician claims	Care provided by physicians, nurse practitioners, physician assistants, and other allied health professionals (ie, physical and occupational therapists) not covered in an institutional claim	Procedure level	• Unique member identifier
			• Unique encounter identifier
			• Service date
			• Diagnoses
			• Procedure
			• Costs
			  ○ Total
			  ○ Patient
			  ○ Insurer/employer

Prescription claims	Filled prescriptions	Prescription level	• Unique member identifier
			• Unique claim identifier
			• Service date
			• Drug name/identifier
			• Dose
			• Days supplied
			• Costs
			  ○ Total
			  ○ Patient
			  ○ Insurer/employer

be conducted and the generalizations made. For example, it would be impossible to conduct a study determining whether users of a certain asthma medication had fewer emergency room visits without both the prescription and medical claims. Following is a brief overview of the enrollment file, the 2 separate databases used to capture medical claims, and the prescription claims database.

Enrollment File

The enrollment file is the insurer's record of who has coverage at any given time. Whenever an enrollee or qualified dependent joins or leaves a plan, it is reflected in the enrollment file. As one can easily understand, it is important for the insurer to know if a patient had coverage at the time of their medical care so that they do not pay for charges incurred when the patient was not covered. Patients in the enrollment file have a unique identifier that is also present on all of their claims. The enrollment file contains demographic information such as name, age, sex, and address for each patient. The file also contains information on the plan in which the patient is enrolled. Although the researcher may not receive all of the information contained in the enrollment file (because personal data such as patient name and address are often de-identified), the unique identifier and dates of coverage are critically important to most database research because they allow all of an individual's claims to be linked and to account for gaps in coverage.

Medical Claims Databases

Medical claims are usually collected in 2 distinct databases. The first includes institutional or hospital claims, and the second includes claims from health care professionals (eg, physicians, physical therapists). The reason for having 2 distinct databases is based in part on how the care for each is reimbursed. Institutional care is generally reimbursed for an episode of care (eg, a single reimbursement for a hospital stay), whereas most professional service is reimbursed based on procedures (eg, an office visit, a therapy session, a surgical procedure). Although the databases are distinct, there are also similarities. In both cases, the claim is generally filed after the care has been provided (although some procedures require preapproval). At the time the care is provided, the physician or other provider indicates what care was provided either on a standardized form or chart. From that information, a professional medical coder and/or billing specialist prepares and submits the claim to the insurer for payment.

Institutional/Hospital Claims

When a patient is admitted to a hospital, many aspects are involved in the patient's care (eg, nursing care, meals and room, medications). Led by Medicare, insurers have moved away from paying for each element of care separately. Instead, most hospital care is reimbursed based on the primary reason for the admission. The diagnosis-related group (DRG) system classifies admissions into 1 of approximately 500 groups (eg, DRG 489 corresponds with pneumonia and DRG 89 with congestive heart failure). Insurers are able to prospectively negotiate reimbursement levels for each group. As a result, hospital claims data do not include details on all elements of the care provided. Generally, a single hospital or institutional claim will included a unique claim identifier, an institution identifier, the admission and discharge dates, the DRG or Major Diagnostic Category codes for the diagnoses associated with the admission, codes for the procedures performed during the admission, and a single charge and reimbursement amount for the entire stay. The hospital claim will not include care provided by physicians. This care will show up in the professional claims database.

Professional Claims

Professional or provider claims include all care provided by physicians, nurse practitioners, physician assistants, and other allied health professionals (ie, physical and occupational therapists). Unlike institutional claims, each professional claim is tied to a single event or procedure so that a visit to a physician's office that includes a blood draw and a minor medical procedure may include several claims. There would be a claim for the actual office visit, one or more for the laboratory work, and a separate claim for the procedure. The American Medical Association has developed the Current Procedural Terminology (CPT) codes as a way of organizing all medical, surgical, and diagnostic services. The CPT codes are used by the insurer to determine the reimbursement to the provider. In addition to the CPT codes, professional claims include a unique claim identifier, a provider identifier, the date of service, a diagnosis code, and information on the charge and reimbursement. As of 2008, pharmacists have 3 CPT codes, exclusively for the profession.

Prescription Claims

Although there is some difference between the 2 types of medical claims, there is an even greater difference between medical and prescription claims databases. Unlike medical claims, which are generally not submitted until after the care has been provided, prescription claims are usually adjudicated prior to the dispensing of the prescription. This requires an automated system to handle a high number of transactions instantly. As a result of this high volume of relatively inexpensive transactions, most prescription claims are handled by PBMs rather than by the insurer. The information required to process a prescription claim dictates the data captured. Prescription claims generally contain the following information: a unique claim identifier, identifier for the prescriber and dispenser, the date of service, information about the prescription (eg, drug name, National Drug Code [NDC] number, dosage, route of administration, days of supply), and the charge and reimbursement amount (including the amount to be collected from the patient). Although it is changing, prescription claims generally do not include information about the diagnosis or reason for the prescription, which can limit their usefulness.

■ What Are the Advantages and Disadvantages of Using Claims Databases?

Using claims databases for research will not be appropriate in all cases. Motheral and Fairman[1] have previously described some of the advantages and disadvantages to using this data source. In this section, we will highlight some of the key advantages and disadvantages of using these data.

Advantages

The primary advantages of using claims databases (or any existing data source) relative to primary, prospective data collection are related to the ease and costs of data collection. Primary data collection for an RCT can be very costly and time consuming. Imagine collecting data on patients with a rare condition for an RCT. It will likely involve multiple sites (with the accompanying training costs) to identify a sufficient number of patients. Recruitment may take a couple of months or up to several years. Once identified, patients will have to agree to be participants and someone will have to monitor and record the data over time. Assuming you desired a year of follow-up, you would have to have all of the data collected for a year after the last patient was enrolled. What if you wanted 5 years of follow-up?

With claims databases, it is not uncommon to have access to 5 or more years' worth of data on over a million patients at the time that you receive approval for the study. In other words, you have almost instant access to a huge patient population for considerably less money in most cases. Why is this advantageous to health outcomes researchers? Think about some of the questions we want to answer. Does prolonged exposure to Drug X improve long-term outcomes? How do patients with this rare condition react to Drug Y? These and other research questions that require long exposure or follow-up times or deal with rare events cannot be practically studied with RCTs or other prospective methods. The real advantage of these data sources is access to large sample sizes over a long duration at a relatively low cost.

The next big advantage of claims databases relative to most RCTs is the generalizability of the results. Most RCTs are restrictive in their study populations and very carefully control patient exposure to the medications of interest. For example, they may restrict the study population to patients with no comorbid conditions, or they may use blood tests or other checks of patient compliance. Unfortunately, patients in the real world are noncompliant and may have multiple comorbidities. This limits the generalizability of RCTs because patients are not treated in controlled, ideal conditions. Studies using claims databases have the advantage of comparing patients under real-world conditions. Although this may make it more difficult to determine a true relationship between an exposure and an outcome, it does make the result more generalizable when one is found.

Disadvantages

The biggest disadvantage of using medical and prescription claims data in research is that the data were not collected for research purposes. This means that it is not possible to employ true experimental design. The researcher does not have any control over a subject's exposure to the intervention, which means that exposure cannot be randomized. This means that there may be meaningful differences between the study arms not only in the number of subjects exposed, but also with regard to factors that may confound the results. Later in the chapter, we will discuss some of the quasi-experimental designs used to address such limitations.

As discussed earlier, the primary role of claims databases is to allow for the processing of efficient financial transactions. This means that the variables in the databases are generally limited to just those elements necessary to complete the financial transaction. Because the need for clinical information is limited, another major disadvantage of using claims databases is the lack of important clinical information. Claims databases will almost never include laboratory values or the results of a diagnostic test or procedure. As a result, it may be difficult to determine clinical outcome from a claim, and in some cases, it may be difficult to determine whether a patient actually has the disease of interest. A claim to rule out a condition will still include the diagnosis on the claim. For that reason, researchers generally require multiple claims on different dates to positively identify a patient as having the disease of interest.

Another disadvantage of claims databases is that they are only as good as the data entered into them. Although the data are generally valid and reliable, there are a few factors that can affect the accuracy of the coding on which most database research relies and can lead to misclassification bias. First, coding by its very nature requires the distillation of whatever care is provided into a series of predefined diagnoses and procedures. As one might imagine, it can be extremely difficult to adequately code an extremely difficult episode of care. The second coding issue relates back to the primary use of the information. Both the provider and the insurer have a financial incentive to select certain codes for an episode of care.

A provider has an incentive to "up code" or include all of a patient's diagnoses and to choose a higher reimbursing procedure code if there is a choice between multiple similar codes. Likewise, the payer has an incentive to "down code" or reimburse for the lesser code. As a result, it is not always possible to definitively determine the exact care received or to compare between providers. Efforts have been made to improve the transparency in coding, which limits this issue.

The final issue that impacts the accuracy of databases is that they may not capture all care, including interventions that a patient receives. For example, if a patient goes to a pharmacy and pays cash for her generic angiotensin-converting enzyme inhibitor without having the pharmacy process the claim, the claim will never appear in the database. As a result, the patient adherence may be underestimated. Also over-the-counter (OTC) medications are rarely captured in a claims database, and medication samples are rarely captured as well. Another concern is for patients covered under multiple insurance plans (eg, Medicare and a supplemental private plan) whose care may not show up in a database if it was covered under the other plan.

The last major disadvantage of using claims databases in research is related to the generalizability of the results. As discussed earlier, the external validity of claims-based research is generally greater than for an RCT, but that does not mean they can always be generalized to all populations. Most claims databases in the United States come from private insurers and represent patients with employer-based coverage. As a result, the populations tend to be younger, healthier, and of a higher socioeconomic status than the general public. This may limit the generalizability of the results to patient populations who are older or do not have the same access to care (eg, Medicaid and Medicare recipients). In addition, many of the databases reflect a limited geographical region, which may further limit their generalizability.

■ Types of Studies Conducted with Medical and Prescription Claims Databases

Because of their large size, reflection of actual care patterns, and relatively low cost, databases are used in a wide variety of studies. The following are the most common applications, and they build on a recent review of the uses of databases in epidemiologic research.[2]

Utilization Studies

Claims databases are well suited for studies examining utilization of a drug or procedure. Studies showing the prevalence, incidence, duration, and variability of utilization can be used for assessing quality and variations in care. Utilization information that would be difficult to collect via patient recall can be taken directly from a claims database. For example, researchers using prescription claims data for 9 million eligible members looked at the utilization of rosiglitazone and pioglitazone at a time when there were announcements about public safety concerns for these medications related to their safety.[3]

Adverse Event Studies

Studies using claims databases can be particularly useful for assessing adverse events because of their ability to follow large numbers of subjects over extended periods of time. This allows for the detection of rare events that may take years to be observed in smaller more controlled populations. For example, researchers using claims databases were able to examine the effect of antiepileptic drug substitutions on events requiring emergency room visits and hospitalizations.[4]

Comparative Effectiveness

As mentioned earlier, one of the advantages of these studies is their generalizability due to the fact that the data come from real-world utilization. This allows studies using claims databases to look at effectiveness rather than efficacy. Because they can compare multiple active treatments, claims database research is the most practical option for comparative effectiveness research, which will be discussed more in Chapter 14. A recent example compared the effectiveness of different β-adrenergic antagonists on patient mortality for patients with heart failure.[5]

Health Policy Research

Claims databases are commonly used to evaluate how changes in policy at either the national or insurance plan level impact clinical and economic outcomes. Their longitudinal nature, capture of actual utilization, and flexibility in selecting control groups make these databases ideal for evaluating the effects of policy changes. For example, researchers using prescription claims data to look at a switch in insurance plan design from a flat copayment (eg, a set dollar amount) to coinsurance (eg, a percentage of payment) found that the switch moderated the growth in overall prescription costs and prescription utilization.[6]

How Does One Get Access to Medical and Prescription Claims Databases?

Earlier, we stated that one big advantage of using claims databases is that they provide relatively inexpensive access to a large number of subjects. This does not mean that it will be easy or free for most researchers to access the data. In most cases, someone "owns" the data, and using it for research purposes requires the owner providing access to the database. In this section, we will discuss some of the primary sources of claims databases, as well as some of the issues to consider when accessing them.

Most of the studies conducted in the United States use private insurer data. Many insurers employ their own outcomes researchers to conduct studies that are of particular interest to the insurer or their clients. Often, this research is also of interest to the larger community and finds its way into publication. For these researchers, access to their own claims data is not an issue. Unfortunately, most researchers do not have such easy access to data. For others with no such access to internal claims data, there are 2 primary approaches to obtaining claims data.

The first approach is to purchase the data directly from the owner of the data. There are a number of companies in the United States that maintain proprietary research databases (eg, Thomson Healthcare's MarketScan). These claims databases generally contain individual-level claims from a number of employers or insurers. The biggest advantage of these databases is that they are intended for research purposes so the data have been cleaned and formatted for ease of use. However, because these databases are proprietary products, they are relatively expensive. For that reason, pharmaceutical companies or other sources fund most of the studies that use these databases. Furthermore, researchers get access only to the data they purchase, which means they may have a limited number of years. In addition, the researcher may have limited information on elements of the insurance plans included which may affect their research. For example, did a plan implement a prior authorization program for proton pump inhibitors (PPIs)? If so, when did the program start, and what would that mean for a study looking at PPI utilization?

The other approach researchers have for accessing private insurance claims databases is to obtain them directly from the insurer or PBM. If successful, the data can be obtained at little or no cost. That said, it is difficult to obtain data in this manner. Most of these organizations are very reluctant to share their data with researchers they do not know. It is almost always necessary to develop or have an existing relationship with someone at the insurer prior to obtaining data. Even then, it is unlikely that a researcher will be given free access to the data. Generally, a researcher will have to propose a project which has some inherent value to the organization before the organization is willing to share the data. Even then, the data provided will be probably the minimum necessary to complete the project. In addition, most organizations do not consider outside research a priority, so it may take time to get the data, and the researcher may not have much control over the format in which the data are received. Finally, there may be limitations on what data are accessible. For example, the insurer may only have the past 3 years' worth of data available or may not have prescription data for some portion of the covered lives.

Regardless of which of the 2 approaches is used, access to the data will include some restrictions. Researchers will have to comply with the Health Insurance Portability and Accountability Act's Privacy Rule (HIPAA). Depending on what protected health information (PHI) the researcher needs, this is likely include a review by the institutional review board (IRB) and the creation of a data use agreement between the insurer and the researcher. Using de-identified data allows a researcher to use data without restriction under the Privacy Rule. The National Institutes of Health provides a detailed overview of the requirements for using PHI and of what identifiers need to be removed for a database to be considered de-identified.[7]

One final consideration for the researcher is some of the information contained in a database is proprietary and may not be available to the researcher. For example, an insurer may be unwilling to share both the amount charged and the amount paid for a claim because it may allow for the determination of reimbursement rates or discounts. Because this information is critical to the competitiveness of an organization, it is unlikely they would be willing to release that information.

Despite the difficulties, limitations, and restrictions associated with accessing medical and prescription claims databases, these data sources are available to the industrious researcher. Although the restrictions and limitations of the data will make some research impossible or impractical, there is still an almost endless number of studies that can be conducted with these databases for the researcher who understands the methods required for conducting a study using claims data.

■ Developing a Study That Uses a Claims Database

To reflect the uniqueness and peculiarities of each database, it has been said that if you have seen one claims database, you have seen one claims database. The same can be said about studies using claims data. Although there are some common methodologies in the development of these studies, every study will be different and require a unique combination of study design, assumptions (ie, inclusion criteria), and analytic methods. At times, this may involve as much art as science, which is why it always critical for researchers to be transparent in their methodology and to clearly state any and all assumptions they have used. This section will provide some of the basics in conducting database studies, but it is by no means a comprehensive guide. New researchers are encouraged to seek out additional training on the methods or collaborate with more seasoned investigators to further develop their skills.

Study Design

As discussed earlier, the biggest disadvantage of using retrospective claims data in research is that the subjects and subsequent intervention(s) cannot be randomized. This means that database research cannot use true experimental design. In place of the true experimental design, researchers must use quasi-experimental designs, which are study designs that share many similarities with experimental design. Most importantly, these designs allow for the identification of an independent variable that can be used to group patients by exposure status (eg, statin use) to determine the effect on the dependent or outcome variable (eg, number of cardiac events). Because there is no randomization, quasi-experimental designs cannot eliminate the possibility of confounding bias, which limits the ability to draw causal influences. Statistical and design techniques are available to control this bias.

Study Types

The two most commonly used designs are the cohort and case-control study. In both study designs, the intent is to show whether prior exposure affects the outcome of interest. In classic epidemiologic studies, the cohort study is considered a prospective study. Patients are identified based on exposure status (ie, smoking status) and then followed forward in time to see if they differ in the outcome of interest (ie, diagnosis of lung cancer). The case-control study is a retrospective study where patients with the outcome of interest are identified (cases) and then matched to patients in the same population without the outcome of interest (controls). Then the researcher looks back to identify exposure status. Because all database studies are conducted using retrospective data, the practical application for outcomes research is slightly different. Simply put, the major difference between the designs is whether the study population is divided by exposure status or outcome status. Chapter 9 will further describe the use of patient reported data.

Claims databases can also be used for descriptive studies or cross-sectional studies. Until now, we have focused on experimental or analytic study designs—that is, studies that consider the time perspective or whether the exposure occurred prior to the outcome. Claims data can also be used to show a correlation between an exposure and an outcome at a given point in time without concern for which came first. This is obviously a less powerful study design, but it does still have practical applications, especially for hypothesis generation.

Eligibility and Exclusion Criteria

As previously mentioned, an advantage of database studies is their external validity or generalizability to the overall populations. This can also serve as a challenge to the researcher when one considers the potential for bias. Therefore, it is often advisable for the researcher to establish inclusion and/or exclusion criteria for entry into the study. Although the criteria will vary significantly from study to study, the following are commonly used criteria. Subjects who are not continuously enrolled with the insurer for the entire duration of the database or at least a minimum period of time (ie, 24 months) are often excluded because it is not possible to completely capture their utilization. Likewise, many studies will exclude patients 65 or older because it is likely that they also have Medicare coverage.

Many studies will also include only incident exposure or outcomes. For example, a study looking at the effect of the duration of statin therapy on preventing cardiac events may exclude subjects who had a statin claim within the first 6 months because it would not be possible to determine the length of therapy that occurred prior to the first date covered in the database. Finally, researchers may simplify their studies by excluding subjects with known confounding conditions, especially those that cannot be well-controlled for statistically. An example would be to exclude all subjects with diabetes from a study where the severity of diabetes would influence the outcome. Because it is difficult to assess the severity of a disease from diagnosis or procedure codes, the researcher may be better off excluding those patients and recognizing it as a limitation of their study.

Variable Identification

This leads directly to the next issue in conducting a study with a claims database. How does a researcher identify the outcome, the exposure, and potential confounders using a claims database? Codes are proxies for actual diagnosis (International Classification of Diseases, 9th Revision, Clinical Modification [ICD9-CM]), procedures (CPT), or medications (NDC or Generic Product Identifier [GPI]). Determining a subject's true illness and treatment from the codes can pose a sizeable challenge. In some cases, it is relatively easy to identify the condition of interest from a well-defined diagnosis code (eg, ICD9-CM 038.12 for methicillin-resistant *Staphylococcus aureus* septicemia) or range of codes (eg, ICD9-CM 410.00 to 410.92 for acute myocardial infarction). On other occasions, researchers may need to use clinical judgment to exclude certain codes within a range because they do not reflect the condition of interest. It is also not uncommon for researcher to use a combination of diagnosis, procedure, and drug codes to identify all cases of a particular condition.

Researchers must also make assumptions when defining the condition of interest and determining what codes to include. For example, if it is important to include all claims for acute interstitial nephritis (ICD9-CM 580.89), which is often misdiagnosed and therefore miscoded, the researcher may have to include other less specific codes (ICD9-CM 584.9 [acute renal failure, unspecified]). Once again, researchers are encouraged to be transparent with the selected codes and the methods used to select them.

Index Dates

A final consideration for the design of database research is how to deal with date issues. Of particular concern are issues related to the length of exposure and follow-up, and index dates. Both issues require the researcher to standardize dates to allow for appropriate analysis. With regard to length of exposure and follow-up, the researcher must ensure there was ample time to detect exposure prior to identification of an outcome and time to detect an outcome after the exposure. Imagine the potential problems with a study looking at the effect of adherence to low-dose inhaled corticosteroid therapy on asthma-related emergency room visits where one subject was diagnosed with asthma and filled their first prescription a month before the end of the study period, whereas another subject had 24 months of follow-up after their diagnosis. Would it be fair to compare either the adherence or outcomes for those 2 subjects? For this reason, researchers often standardize their study period so that everyone has the same opportunity for exposure and outcome.

Sometimes, researchers will use a specific date range (eg, January 1, 2008 through December 31, 2008) for their study period, but they may also use a period of time around an index event. Here the researcher identifies the date of some event (eg, drug-eluting stent insertion) or exposure (eg, first prescription fill) and then requires subjects to have a certain amount of claim history before and after this index date. The index date allows for subjects' exposure status to be compared over certain time periods (eg, 1-year adherence) even when the initial exposure dates vary. It also allows for the evaluation of time-dependent outcomes (eg, time until inpatient readmission).

Analysis of Claims Data

Confounding Variables

As discussed earlier, for the types of quasi-experimental studies conducted using claims databases to address issues of causality, they must control for the presence of confounders. These are factors related to both the exposure and outcome of interest which may affect the relationship between the two (eg, older patients are more likely to be taking a β-blocker and to be hard of hearing, so a study looking at the relationship between these factors would want to control for the subjects' age). Although it is virtually impossible for these studies to completely eliminate confounding, they can use exclusion criteria, matching, and/or statistical techniques to control for it. For a researcher to control for potential confounders, she must first identify them. For this reason, it is important for researchers to develop an a priori model including all of the factors that could influence the relationship between the exposure and the outcome.

Exclusion criteria and matching based on a potential confounder (eg, age) are relatively straightforward and will not be discussed further in this chapter. The most common technique used to control for confounding is the use of multivariable regression models.

Regression Models

The nature of the outcome variable will determine the most appropriate regression model (ie, linear regression for a continuous variable, logistic regression for dichotomous outcome, or proportional hazards regression for survival data). Selection of the most appropriate model often requires consultation with a biostatistician. Regardless of the model used, all of the models attempt to estimate the effect of the exposure on the outcome after controlling for the effect of the potential confounders. Regression analyses are only as good as the variables tested, which includes the completeness of the model considered, which factors could actually be collected from the databases, and the accuracy of the data. That is why it is imperative that researchers explain their assumptions and decisions for each of the factors selected.

Interpretation of Findings

Because it is unlikely a researcher will ever be able to completely control for all potential confounders, care must be taken when interpreting the results of any claims-based research. With adequate care and transparency, it is possible to draw conclusions from these studies, but most researchers will stop short of stating certain causality based on the results of any single observational study. Once more, researchers should clearly state any and all limitations with their data that could affect their results. This allows the consumer of the research to consider how those factors may have affected the results and ultimately whether they choose to accept the researchers' conclusions.

■ Mini-Case

As a means of considering how claims databases can be used in health outcomes research, let's consider the following case. A physician in your clinic mentions that she had recently seen a relatively healthy patient with mild renal injury consistent with acute interstitial nephritis (AIN). She was not sure of the cause of the injury, but knew several classes of medications had been linked to AIN. The only medication this particular patient was taking was from a widely used class. The class was generally considered safe and had even had some lesser used members of the class approved for OTC use. At her request, you did a literature search that only turned up a handful of case reports suggesting a link between the drug class and AIN. Unsatisfied with the available evidence, you begin to ask yourself whether there is some way to better answer the question. Given that the outcome seems rare and the drugs have been on the market for quite some time, you recognize that an RCT is probably impractical. Would this study be a candidate for a claims database study? Why or why not?

After contacting a colleague at a managed care organization, you are granted access to their data to study the possible relationship between use of the medication class and AIN. He says you can have access to data on 800,000 members for the past 5 years, but you need to let him know what data sets and variables you need. Although excited, you are also concerned about conducting a methodologically sound study. His question opens up several questions. How will you define exposure? How will you define and identify AIN? Are there other factors that could influence the relationship between the medication's use and AIN? Which databases will you need?

Things are moving pretty fast now. After identifying the data required to conduct the study, you received approval from your institution's IRB, submitted your official data request to the managed care organization, and received the de-identified data. Now that you have the data, in addition to being overwhelmed by the size of the data set, you are in the process of determining which subjects were exposed to the medications class, which had the outcome of interest, and which confounders are present. A colleague sees your list of potential confounders and wonders how you will control for them all. What are the possible methods to control for confounding?

It has taken longer than anticipated, but you have finally completed your analysis. Even after controlling for all of the confounders, a statistically significant relationship between the medication class and AIN exists. As you begin writing the manuscript, you begin to consider what your results mean. Do the results of your study confirm that exposure to this medication class causes AIN? Why or why not?

■ Summary

Medical and prescription claims databases provide researchers with a wealth of existing data that can be used to conduct outcomes research. Although they will never replace prospectively conducted RCTs for determining causality, these studies do play an important role in advancing knowledge and influencing decision making. The large study population and the retrospective nature of the data make these data sources particularly useful for the rare outcomes and long follow-up times which are impractical for prospective studies. As the methodologies for conducting claims-based research improve and the technology for linking claims to clinical information becomes more widespread, many of the concerns with this type of research will be lessened, and the use and value of these databases will become even more widespread.

■ References

1. Motheral BR, Fairman KA. The use of claims databases for outcomes research: rationale, challenges and strategies. *Clin Ther*. 1997;19:346–366.
2. Schneeweiss S, Avorn J. A review of uses of health care utilization databases for epidemiologic research on therapeutics. *J Clin Epidemiol*. 2005;58:323–337.

3. Starner CI, Schafer JA, Heaton AH, Gleason PP. Rosiglitazone and pioglitazone utilization from January 2007 through May 2008 associated with five risk-warning events. *J Manag Care Pharm.* 2008;14:523–531.

4. Rascati KL, Richards KM, Johnsrud MT, Mann TA. Effects of antiepileptic drug substitutions on epileptic events requiring acute care. *Pharmacotherapy.* 2009;29:769–774.

5. Go AS, Yang J, Gurwitz JH et al. Comparative effectiveness of different beta-adrenergic antagonists on mortality among adults with heart failure in clinical practice. *Arch Intern Med.* 2008;168:2415–2421.

6. Klepser DG, Huether JR, Handke LJ, Williams CE. Effect on drug utilization and expenditures of a cost-share change from copayment to coinsurance. *J Manag Care Pharm.* 2007;13:765–777.

7. National Institutes of Health. How can covered entities use and disclose protected health information for research and comply with the Privacy Rule? http://privacyruleandresearch.nih.gov/pr_08.asp. Accessed May 23, 2011.

Uses of Real-World Data in Evidence Development

Carl V. Asche, PhD

Carl V. Asche, PhD

Learning Objectives

- Describe the uses of patient registries in evidence development.
- Provide an understanding of creating, operating, and evaluating registries.
- Discuss motivation of measuring patient-reported outcomes in a patient registry.

■ Introduction

Efficacy and safety are presumed from randomized controlled trials (RCTs). However, these data are from only on a very small portion of patients and generally not representative of the real world due to clinical protocol criteria. For example, most patients with comorbidities are excluded, and the impact of patient compliance is often not captured. Payers want to now know about value and comparative effectiveness (is another option better than the currently available alternatives) in real-world settings. These are the data they need to decide whether drug reimbursement is warranted versus what is already being used to treat a particular disease.

The learning objectives of this chapter are to be able to describe advantages and disadvantages of observational studies using real-world data compared with RCTs and to describe data sources available for health outcomes studies and compare claims databases with electronic health records (EHRs). This chapter focuses on RCTs versus real-world study types and observational studies, data sources for observational studies, and claims data versus EHRs.

■ Study Types

Whereas descriptive studies aim to describe as closely as possible what has happened without interpretation or explanation, the objective of explanatory studies is to understand and use the new knowledge for further insights; thus, explanatory studies are often preferred by clinicians. The 2 main types of explanatory studies are experimental controlled studies and observational studies. Experimental studies compare an observation of an intervention group with those of a control group and thereby try to understand a path or mechanism of action. Observational studies also try to understand causes and mechanisms by observing the course of a development, its normal or typical variations, and changes over time in a natural setting (eg, normal clinical practice).

Prospective Explanatory Studies: Process and Characteristics

In RCTs, patients are enrolled and then randomized to the treatment. Patients in prospective observational trials are managed based on the doctor's decision according to standard practice. These patients are enrolled in the trial if they fit the inclusion criteria. It is important to compare the characteristics of RCTs to observational studies. When dealing with bias, RCTs attempt to reduce it by keeping the physician and patient out of the treatment selection process. Observational studies contain bias because the treatment study occurs like a normal situation, where control is minimized. Patients who discontinue their medication(s) are either excluded, as in RCTs, or have the option to switch treatment. To determine which patients should be used in the study, RCTs gather a treatment group designed to reduce patient variability, whereas observational studies include, or exclude, patients based on disease criteria and type of treatment at the start. RCTs, by nature, contain artificially homogenous patient populations to improve the level of effect detection. Observational studies contain heterogeneous (eg, similar) patient populations that are more likely to reflect a real-world practice in that there is variance in the patients.

RCTs have strict care protocols and few choices of alternate drugs to limit confounding factors. They also have the highest standard of care due to tight supervision, high control levels, and various tests. Observational studies have a low level of interference with treatment in order to mimic real-life situations and are considered "care as usual," resulting in the typical standard of care. RCTs end at objectively measurable clinical end points (eg, efficacy), whereas observational studies simply have outcomes, which are more subjective (eg, effectiveness). Thus, RCT results are measured in terms of efficacy, whereas the results from observational studies are measured in terms of effectiveness.

Gold Standard for Health Care: RCTs

RCTs are the "gold standard" or benchmark for clinical decision making in health care. One of the defining properties of an RCT is that it starts the experiment with "equal" experimental groups. The way to create this equality is through randomization. The results of RCTs are considered to be evidence level A (the best). However, RCTs can take a long time to complete and are usually very expensive. They are driven by a protocol, and the protocol may be different from the way patients are treated under natural conditions. Multiple types of controls can be used, including placebos or previous standard therapies.

■ Which Study Type Should Be Used and When?

The challenge is deciding which study type to use to answer the research question. RCTs are used to prove clinical efficacy and safety, defined by the following question: Can the treatment maintain efficacy and safety under these conditions in this patient population? These data will have to be validated in real-world observational studies once the product is used by a broader patient population.[1] The clinical effectiveness is analyzed in observational studies. These studies can either be prospective, using registries and patient-reported outcomes (PROs), or retrospective, using analyses of EHRs and claims data.

■ Types of Real-World Studies

Real-world data can be retrieved in various types of databases. Some of these databases are easily accessible and well known, whereas others only exist for a limited time or for a closely defined population. Each of the potential sources for data has its advantages and limitations. The knowledge of these is important to be able to use appropriate data for each of the questions to be addressed in real-world data studies.[1] The quality of the data will critically impact the quality of the research.

Supplements to RCTs

RCTs can be supplemented to collect additional data on resource use, cost, or PROs such as satisfaction or quality of life. These are not typical measures for RCTs, and usually the number of patients is not sufficient to get significant results on these secondary end points. Often the duration of the RCTs is too limited to reveal relevant outcomes data, and the determination of the treatment path by the study protocol will limit the relevance of the results for the actual use of the intervention in real life.

For example, quality of life or patient satisfaction may be perceived differently under the stricter conditions of the RCT then under the normal treatment pathway. Similarly, cost impact will be different in the RCT situation because the treatment is determined by the study protocol, which may include measures that are not usually used.[1]

Observational Studies

Observational studies draw data from larger patient populations. The design of observational studies can be based on observation of a cohort or fixed patient population over a longer time frame, for example, all inhabitants of a village or all patients diagnosed with diabetes between 2000 and 2002 in a database. Alternatively, a case-control study compares patients with a disease or who received a specific treatment with a matched group of patients without the disease or who did not receive that treatment or received an alternative treatment. Because of the observational approach of treatment as it is applied in normal practice, the cost of observational studies is usually much lower than the cost of RCTs.

There are also disadvantages with observational studies. Because of the observational approach, it is often assumed that there is a selection bias of patients. If there are 2 different therapies available, it is highly probable that the decision to use one therapy over the other is made in a systematic manner and leads to differences between the treatment group and the comparator group. For example, if one of the drugs is frequently accompanied by diarrhea, the doctor may not use this drug to treat a patient who is suffering from bowel problems. For the same reason as biased patient selection, treatment effects may be more expressed in an observational study than they would be in the RCT approach.[2] Because observational studies, especially long-term studies, involve the collection and analysis of large data sets, they may result in relatively high cost and complex analysis protocols. For the decision maker, the use of observational evidence may seem to be less reliable because there is still a lack of standardization in methods of evaluation and interpretation.

Patient Registries

Patient registries are prospective collections of data across a disease state or of patients who are receiving specific therapies. Registries provide baseline data for cost of illness analyses, economic modeling, and future study designs. Registries have the advantage that they are built specifically for a disease and therefore collect the appropriate information that is needed to answer research questions. In decision making, they may also be used to confirm conclusions drawn from RCTs, when there is doubt about the relevance of the RCT data for real-life situations. Patient registries are usually not used to compare therapies or to identify opportunities for treatment improvement.[3]

Patient-Reported Outcomes

A PRO is a measurement of any aspect of a patient's health status that comes directly from the patient, without the interpretation of the patient's responses by a physician or anyone else.[4] PROs are measured through questionnaires, surveys, diaries, and interviews. PROs are observations from the perspective of the patient. Examples of PROs are quality-of-life data, measures of productivity, and patient preferences.

PRO instruments, such as surveys, can be either disease-specific or general, whereby specific instruments often have a higher resolution in disease-specific domains, but do not allow for comparisons across different disease states. Disease-specific scales are useful to study the impact and mechanism of a specific therapy on a specific aspect of a disease. However, for reimbursement decisions, the decision makers usually request the use of general questions to enable them to assess the results compared with other therapy types in other disease areas.

Different types of scales can be used to measure quality of life. Examples include global assessment scales and visual analog scales; the latter is a continuous scale between 0, indicating death, and 1, indicating best possible quality of life. Quality-of-life data are usually complimentary to other data or evidence.

The importance of quality-of-life data is recognized by regulatory agencies, formularies, physicians, and patients. To clarify the role of patient-reported data in the drug approval process and to refine standards for PRO instrument development, in February 2006, the US Food and Drug Administration issued guidance on PRO measures. The National Cancer Institute (NCI) responded to the guidance by sponsoring the NCI PROs Assessment in Cancer Trials conference in September 2006. They decided that the patient's own account should be considered the gold standard.[5]

Data Sources: Retrospective Data Analysis

Retrospective data analysis studies existing data without interfering with the treatment. The data have usually been collected for different purposes, and the analysis is guided and documented by an analysis plan. Previously collected data (RCTs, administrative databases, health records) are retrospectively analyzed following an analysis plan. The type of data is fixed, and no additional data can be requested. These data analyses are created primarily for insurance claims for reimbursement. People or organizations who usually request these types of analyses are the federal government, state governments, and private health care insurers. Retrospective database analyses use existing databases to analyze treatment patterns and treatment impact in a given population.

Treatment codes can be used to retrieve patient information. For example, diabetic patients may be identified by selecting all patients in the database who receive any type of antidiabetic treatment. The subgroup that also suffers from hypertension can be identified by selecting all patients receiving antidiabetic and antihypertensive treatment.[6] Adherence to the treatment can be measured by following the number and regularity of refills for a specific patient. Data are usually collected directly during patient visits. Thus, they reflect the direct observation and the management pattern of the provider.

Retrospective data analyses are relatively inexpensive and can cover large patient populations over long periods of time and, for example, analyze the prescribing patterns in such populations. Typical limitations of retrospective data analyses are a lack of internal validity, caused by incomplete diagnostic information, and variation of compliance in the population, which is not monitored or documented or can only be concluded indirectly.

Another often not obvious confounding factor, which may differ among the study groups, is a lack of external validity. This can be caused by specialization of a database on specific patient populations, plan design, regional treatment patterns (eg, urban vs rural, hospital vs outpatient), and cost differences. It should to be noted that each type of database collects only data that serve the original purpose of creating the database. Claims databases are usually administrative databases and do not include detailed clinical or outcomes data besides major end points like death or disability. Sometimes, there is a great delay of data availability because of the administrative processes.[6]

Electronic Health Records

EHRs are used by clinicians to collect all clinically relevant data. Therefore, they contain diagnostic data, laboratory values, and all relevant clinical measurements, as evaluated in the clinic or office. They are usually up to date and updated during, or shortly after, the patient visit. Thus, they offer rapid access to a broad patient population.[7] Because providers are usually not well networked and generally do not use the same database, patient data are scattered across the universe of their providers. Once patients do not return to a specific provider or leave the hospital, the data are no longer updated. For example, for a study that is designed to analyze the impact of 1 year of treatment throughout the year following this treatment, only patients with at least 1 year of treatment data and 1 year of follow-up data can be included.

The clinicians have some freedom to fill text into the databases, which limits access to this sometimes important information through standardized searches. EHRs reflect the provider view. For example, they will contain prescription orders but will not contain the information on how many prescriptions have actually been filled. Thus, the data will reflect the intention the provider had, but will not show whether the patient followed the recommendations or for how long the patient was compliant with the therapy.

Good Process in Real-World Data

Principles of a good process when using real-world data in decision making were defined by the International Society for Pharmacoeconomics and Outcomes Research (ISPOR), a key organization in the development and formulation of standards and processes in the field of health economics and outcomes research. Of high importance are transparency of process and supporting data. Decision makers need to understand exactly how each step of the model was developed and the bias of all assumptions. The decision and underlying data need to be relevant to the plan's member population. The decision itself needs to be meaningful and just for all members. Ideally the decision-making process should involve all stakeholders.[1]

Noncomparative studies, such as cost-of-illness analysis or trend analysis, may be performed by using patient registries or, sometimes, public health data sources. For health management decisions, EHRs and retrospective data analysis may contain a wealth of additional information.

■ Data Sources: The ISPOR Digest of International Databases

In 2004, the ISPOR Board of Directors expressed interest in providing the ISPOR membership with a central resource to evaluate various data sources. The ISPOR Retrospective Database Special Interest Group Classification of Databases Working Group was tapped to organize and implement this initiative. The working group has since been developing this electronic index (the International Digest of Databases). The Digest now includes 123 databases that list key attributes of health care data from around the world on the ISPOR Web site and is accessible without restriction to the general public. The Digest is grouped by country and allows key word searches and searches by type of database. There is also a comparative feature that will allow the user to view selected databases for review. The initial focus of the Working Group was to classify retrospective data sources through the development and implementation of a data-focused questionnaire. The extended intent of the Working Group is to have an up-to-date, living resource available for all researchers and interested groups to evaluate data sources.

The biggest challenges for the Classification of Databases Working Group were to develop an appropriate questionnaire that would be suitable not only for US-based databases, but also for international database agencies, compile an inclusive list of available national and international data sources, and attempt, to the best of their ability, to get the source agencies to complete the questionnaire. The questionnaire included an additional challenge in the applicability of the current questionnaire to various countries, local markets, and various data sources. To resolve this issue, the Working Group enlisted the help of several international agencies that worked with the working group to design a more appropriate list of questions.

ISPOR has sent invitations to complete the questionnaire to numerous agencies across the globe compiled from members of the Working Group and encouraged the ISPOR membership to either complete the questionnaire if the organization has a health care database or provide names of possible agencies that should be included in the Digest. The response has been encouraging to date, both in completing the questionnaire and interest in using the Digest. Overall, the questionnaire is intended to serve as a tool for researchers and contains the following information:

> **Health care database information:** geographic, hospital, outpatient
> **Database content:** admissions, hospital codes, disease
> **PROs:** symptom response, satisfaction
> **Drug information:** drug name and number of days of supply
> **Insurance information:** drug and medical services coverage

In addition to comments from the ISPOR conference presentations, additional evidence of the utility of the ISPOR Digest has been anecdotally collected over the past few years. The ISPOR Digest has been presented in academic settings for students to understand different types of data (eg, *International Classification of Diseases*, 9th and 10th Revisions), data organizations, and data nuisances for country and regional variations. Several theses have used the ISPOR Digest as a benchmark reference. It has been noted that the ISPOR Digest has saved numerous manufacturer resources (eg, time, budget) by leveraging the Digest as a baseline for types of data and contact information for global data organizations. Of the 123 databases listed in the Digest, databases have been collected from countries in all continents but Africa.

ISPOR has started to build an international repository for databases, which can be accessed through the ISPOR Web site. Each database is described in detail, which allows users to understand the properties of the database, volume of data collected, time frame, and potential value for a specific study. This database is intended to serve as an invaluable source of information for health care outcomes researchers. The Digest benefits not only a multitude of organizations and outcomes researchers around the world, but also health care decision makers and patients, who will ultimately benefit from the information derived from this research. ISPOR is only one possible method for the retrieval and access of databases. Other sources may be government organizations, commercial databases, or organizational databases, for example hospitals or specialist clinics.

■ Real-World Case Studies

We will discuss 3 different case studies of real-world situations. The first is a study of compliance and persistence in hypertension, which has been performed in an administrative claims database called the Integrated HealthCare System. The second is a study of cardio-metabolic risk factors in a primary care setting based on the analysis of EHRs of the General Electric (GE) Centricity database. The third is an assessment of pharmacist chemotherapy preparation cost, which was based on health surveys in 2 academic and 2 community hospitals.

Case Study 1

This study of compliance and persistence in hypertension was performed in an administrative claims database called the Integrated HealthCare System. The data collected allowed for the ability to assess refill rates over time in patients on fixed-dose and free-dose combination therapy, disease state, concomitant medications, and resource use and cost.

As seen in FIGURE 9-1, the data revealed that patients using a fixed-dose combination, in which 2 drugs are in the same dosage form (a pill), have much better persistence (54%) than patients using the same ingredients as a free combination, in which 2 drugs are in separate pills (19%).[8]

In a separate study, a total of 4076 Medicaid recipients from South Carolina who were 18 years of age or older were broken down into 3363 subjects in the fixed-dose combination group and 713 subjects in the free combination group. The mean age of all subjects was 62.2 years; 74.7% were women, and 74.4% were African American.

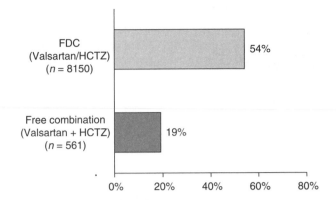

FIGURE 9-1 Case study 1. FDC, fixed-dose combination; HCTZ, hydrochlorothiazide.

Source: Brixner DI, Jackson K, Sheng X, Biskupiak J, Keskinaslan A. Compliance with Multiple Combination Antihypertensive Pharmacotherapy in a Large US Database. *ISPOR European Conference*, Dublin, Ireland, 2007.

The demographics of fixed-dose and free combination groups were similar, although the number receiving fixed-dose combination therapy was nearly 5 times greater.[9] The analysis of total health care cost distribution in both groups showed that patients using the free combination of products incurred almost double the cost of the patients using the fixed-dose combination.

Case Study 2

The second case study describes the cardio-metabolic risk factors in a primary care setting by using EHRs of GE Centricity, which is a large multistate primary care EHR database. The objectives of this study were to define indicators of risk, define the prevalence of individual and cumulative risk, and determine the impact of abdominal obesity on cardio-metabolic risk. The motivation was to validate how well patients at risk can be identified by using the data collected in the EHR.

TABLE 9-1 summarizes the thresholds for determination of the metabolic syndrome for each of the key components including weight, hypertension, lipid characteristics, and diabetes.

Table 9-1	Thresholds for Determination of the Metabolic Syndrome
Risk Factor	Defining Level
Abdominal obesity (waist circumference)	Men: >102 cm (>40 in)
	Women: > 88 cm (>35 in)
High-density lipoprotein cholesterol	Men: <40 mg/dL
	Women: <50 mg/dL
Blood pressure	≥130/≥85 mm Hg
Triglycerides	≥150 mg/dL
Glucose	≥110 mg/dL

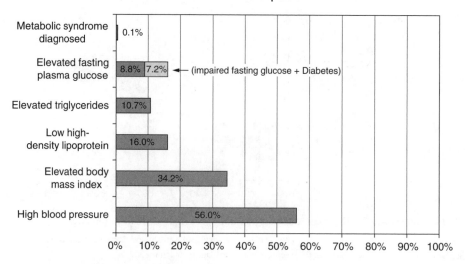

FIGURE 9-2 Cardio-metabolic (CM) risk.

Source: Brixner DI, Said Q, Oderda G, Kirkness C. Assessment of the clinical risk factors for cardiometabolic risk in a national primary care electronic medical record (EMR) database. *Academy of Managed Care Pharmacy 19th Annual Meeting & Showcase,* San Diego, California, 2007.

FIGURE 9-2 depicts the percentage of patients displaying each of the risk factors of interest. Although only 0.1% had an actual diagnosis of metabolic syndrome, 8.8% had an impaired fasting glucose, 10.7% showed elevated triglyceride levels, 16% had low high-density lipoprotein levels, 34.2% an elevated body mass index, and more than half of the patients (56%) had high blood pressure.[10]

Case Study 3

Our third case study is based on surveys and had the objective of determining key cost drivers in the pharmacy for preparing chemotherapy infusions. The breakdown of the key objective is to determine key components of pharmacy-related costs in preparation of chemotherapy infusions, project data from 4 centers to a national insurance claims database, and describe implications of resources and costs on reimbursement policy under the Medicare Modernization Act of 2003. Key cost items included in the analysis are listed in TABLE 9-2, including fixed cost surveys and key cost variables.

This study focused specifically on the pharmacist and technician costs of getting the drug to the patient, exclusive of the drug costs. The purpose was to define the "dispensing fee" associated with oncology drugs. A time-and-motion analysis was performed to understand the resource use of each process step. A time-and-motion study captures the exact activities done in a given period of time. This was done by performing 10 full preparations of infusions and recording the time needed for all the process steps.

Table 9-2	Infusion Preparation Costs for Medicare Patients Receiving Chemotherapy		
		Patients	Infusions
Total*		427,605	2,651,824
Proportion of chemotherapy infusions from top 15 agents		0.66	
Projected Medicare chemotherapy infusions			3,990,495
Number of infusions × calculated cost/infusion from current study		$36.03	$143,777,535
*Medstat MarketScan Medicare and COB Database.			

The results of the simulation were then applied to the total patient population. The number of patients on the drugs studied represented 0.66 of all infusions given in the Medstat Marketscan database. These numbers were then imputed to apply to the national population. As seen in Table 9-2, this resulted in annual preparation costs of $143,777,535 that are not reimbursed by Medicare today.[11]

Conclusions from Real-World Case Studies

Compliance and persistency in hypertension can best be measured in administrative claims databases. EHRs are useful to retrieve clinical data, laboratory values, and diagnostic data. Provider or pharmacist surveys can be used to understand process patterns. The type of database used must be matched up with the specific information needed to answer the research question.

■ Summary

In summary, this chapter defined different study types; compared RCTs to prospective observational studies; defined additional data sources and study types, including patient registries, PROs, claims databases, EHRs, and retrospective data analysis; and discussed 3 different study types that used 3 different sources of data.

■ References

1. Garrison Jr. LP, Neumann PJ, Erickson P, Marshall D, Mullins CD. Using real-world data for coverage and payment decisions: The ISPOR Real-World Data Task Force Report. *Value in Health*. 2007;10:326–335.
2. Tunis SR, Stryer DB, Clancy CM. Practical clinical trials: increasing the value of clinical research for decision making in clinical and health policy. *JAMA*. 2003;290:1624–1632.
3. Hierholzer WJ Jr. Health care data, the epidemiologist's sand: comments on the quantity and quality of data. *Am J Med*. 1991;91:21S–26S.
4. Fowler FJ Jr, Cleary PD, Magaziner J, Patrick DL, Benjamin KL. Methodological issues in measuring patient-reported outcomes: the agenda of the Work Group on Outcomes Assessment. *Med Care*. 1994;32(7 Suppl):JS65–JS76.

5. Trotti A, Colevas AD, Setser A, Basch E. Patient-reported outcomes and the evolution of adverse event reporting in oncology. *J Clin Oncol.* 2007;25:5121–5127.

6. Motheral BR, Fairman KA. The use of claims databases for outcomes research: rationale, challenges and strategies. *Clin Ther.* 1997;19:346–366.

7. Ornstein SM, Oates RB, Fox GN. The computer-based medical record: current status. *J Fam Pract.* 1992;35:556–565.

8. Brixner DI, Jackson K, Sheng X, Biskupiak J, Keskinaslan A. Compliance with Multiple Combination Antihypertensive Pharmacotherapy in a Large US Database. *ISPOR European Conference*, Dublin, Ireland, 2007.

9. Dickson M, Plauschinat CA. Antihypertensive therapy compliance and total cost of care in a Medicaid population: fixed-dose combination versus free combination treatment. *ASHP Summer Meeting.* 2005;62:P71E.

10. Brixner D, Said Q, Kirkness C, et al. Assessment of cardiometabolic risk factors in a national primary care electronic health record database. *Value in Health.* 2006;10:S29-S36.

11. Brixner DI, Oderda GM, Nickman NA, Beveridge R, Jorgenson JA. Documentation of chemotherapy infusion preparation costs in academic- and community-based oncology practices. *J Natl Compr Canc Netw.* 2006;4:197–208.

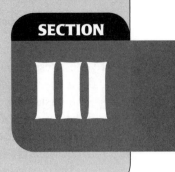
Pharmacoeconomics

Chapter 10 describes two common forms of decision analysis (decision tables and decision trees) used in pharmacoeconomic evaluations. Although data from clinical studies often focus primarily on efficacy and safety, a more realistic picture can be constructed that takes in account not only these parameters, but also other factors that ultimately impact the overall clinical effectiveness of an intervention. Drug acquisition costs alone should not be the only factor considered when selecting medication therapies for either individual patients or populations of patients. Decision analysis allows for a systematic approach to various options and their associated outcomes, given certain variables, leading to the generation of results that can be quantified economically.

Chapter 11 describes what types of economic analysis are available, followed by a description of the elements in economic analysis. Among the elements, types of outcomes, types of costs, and how costs can be determined will be described. Five essential points to consider when conducting economic analysis are described: perspective of the analysis, costs, outcomes, discounting costs and outcomes, and addressing uncertainty. The limitations of economic analysis are also described.

In Chapter 12, cost-of-illness studies and budget impact models are discussed. Cost-of-illness studies describe the total health care costs associated with a specific disease, whereas budget impact models are developed to demonstrate the impact of cost over time for a country, insurance carrier, hospital, or institution for a period of time. How the studies define the health state is critical in representing the disease and the incidence and prevalence of the disease because this is critical to the analysis. Costs associated with a disease state typically include at least 3 types of services: prescriptions, outpatient services, and inpatient services. Chapter 12 also introduces the concepts of presenteeism and absenteeism because they are important in any disease state that interferes with patients' ability to work; these concepts are limited to employer, employee, and societal perspectives.

Chapter 13 further defines cost-benefit analysis, cost-effectiveness analysis, and cost-utility analysis in detail, including the limitations of the analyses. There is also information presented on when each respective analysis is appropriate to use. Also described are quality-adjusted life-years, willingness to pay as an outcome measurement, incremental cost-effectiveness ratio, sensitivity analysis, and cost-effectiveness acceptability curves that can assist both policy makers and clinicians.

The concluding chapter, Chapter 14, provides a look into the future of comparative effectiveness research (CER), which aims to judge relevant treatment options (head-to-head) for a specified condition or disease state at both the individual and population levels. The basic premise behind CER is to provide health care decision makers with data on the outcomes of commonly prescribed therapies to guide the selection of the most effective treatments. Essentially, the value of CER is that it is filling a critical gap in the collective knowledge base by providing data on the success or failure of treatment options administered in actual clinical practice, which will assist consumers, clinicians, purchasers, and policy makers to make informed decisions aimed at improving health care outcomes.

Decision Analysis

George E. MacKinnon III, PhD, RPh, FASHP

Learning Objectives

- Explain the various costs and outcomes assessed in pharmacoeconomic analyses.
- Differentiate between decision tables and decision trees in pharmacoeconomic analyses.
- Understand the primary steps of a pharmacoeconomic analysis.
- Discuss the benefits and limitations of various tools used in pharmacoeconomic analyses.

With the common use of medication formularies by third-party payers (ie, insurers and government plans), health care providers are continually being placed in a position to enforce the decisions and guidelines associated with their implementation in clinical practice. As decision analysis becomes more of a common tool to assist in the decision-making process associated with formulary development and evaluation, it is important that health care providers become familiar with the decision analysis techniques that may have been used to construct a formulary. Although the use of decision analysis for formulary construction is more common in Australia, Canada, and European countries, some insurers and integrated health systems in the United States have adopted these techniques as well.

Historically, health care providers have had an appreciation for both the management and care of individual patients in one setting and from their respective disciplines (eg, medicine, nursing, or pharmacy). Yet increasingly, providers must also be able to oversee the outcomes of care delivered to specific populations of patients in diverse settings, as observed in disease state management for diabetics, anticoagulation, asthmatics, and so on.

Decision analysis is just one of several tools used in pharmacoeconomic evaluations. A benefit associated with decision analysis is that by using data from clinical studies, which often focus primarily on efficacy and safety, a more realistic picture can be constructed that takes into account not only efficacy and safety data, but also other factors that ultimately impact the overall clinical effectiveness of an intervention. As a result, multiple factors can be evaluated, along with their associated costs. For example, a new therapeutic regimen may exhibit 90% efficacy in a highly controlled clinical trial, but when it is used in the general population devoid of such control, this efficacy may diminish because patients may not be compliant with the prescribed regimen and/or they may have other concomitant conditions that can impact the overall clinical effectiveness of the prescribed regimen. Thus, a difference is observed in practice between clinical efficacy and clinical effectiveness.

Decision Analysis Techniques

In the business world, the techniques of decision analysis have been used for many years.[1] In simplistic terms, decision analysis allows for systematic analysis of various options and their associated outcomes, given certain variables, leading to the generation of results that can be quantified.[2] The quantification may result in economic information or criterion ratings. With increased pressure to quantify and justify the value of pharmaceutical products and services, health care providers must understand the various pharmacoeconomic principles and methods used to describe the outcomes (both health-related and economic) associated with the provision of health care services and products. This chapter will describe 2 approaches of decision analysis: decision tables and decision trees.

Decision Tables

A precursor to the decision table is the old paper-and-pencil exercise of listing the "pros and cons" associated between 2 or more choices. Clearly some pros may outweigh the cons and vice versa. In the end, a decision is made by the decision maker(s), but exactly how a selection was made remains unknown. Although this process may be acceptable for individuals, the lack of quantifiable measurement and transparency in making a selection does not sit well when many stakeholders are interested or involved in the decision-making process.

Although similar to the paper-and-pencil exercise of "pros and cons" mentioned earlier, decision tables do require the identification of several alternatives for a stated problem/situation. However, each alternative in the decision table is then evaluated against various criteria that have been identified as being important to various stakeholders. Each criterion receives an assigned weight, which is consistent among all similar criteria of the different alternatives. The total sum of the assigned weights among the criteria must add up to 1.0. The assigned weights essentially prioritize the various criteria to be evaluated in a numerical manner. A criterion that has a greater utility would have a larger numerical value. The foundation of this approach is the multi-attribute utility model.[2]

Additionally, each individual criterion specific to each alternative is given a value rating. This value rating is specific to the alternative and cannot exceed 100 for each criterion being assessed. An alternative that is exceptional may have several scores of 100 for an individual criterion, whereas the criteria for another alternative product could have several values of 0. A final rating is then determined for each criterion by multiplying the assigned weight by the value rating. Each criterion is then added together to determine the overall criteria rating (the range would be 0 to 100).

For example, a comparison is made between products A and B both with equal efficacy for a given disease or condition. The four criteria evaluated for these products are criterion 1 (safety), criterion 2 (efficacy), criterion 3 (dosing convenience), and criterion 4 (drug acquisition cost). Product A is dosed once daily but costs significantly more than product B, which is dosed 3 times daily (thus, a higher value of 75 is assigned to product A for criterion 3). However, product B has a lower drug acquisition cost than product A (thus, a higher value of 100 is assigned to product B for criterion 4). TABLE 10-1 provides an example decision table based on the previously listed conditions. Overall, product B scores higher (77.5) than A (71.5) given the assigned values and weights. Thus, product B is the preferred agent based on this decision table.

Decision Trees

Decision trees provide a graphic representation of each viable alternative selected to be evaluated from beginning to end, depicting the multiple events and sequelae that can result from one or more courses of action (planned or not planned). Essentially, decision

Table 10-1	Example of a Decision Table					
	Value		Assigned Weight		Criterion Rating	
Products	A	B	A	B	A	B
Criterion 1 (safety)	75	100	0.40	0.40	30	40
Criterion 2 (efficacy)	75	75	0.30	0.30	22.5	22.5
Criterion 3 (dosing convenience)	75	25	0.20	0.20	15	5
Criterion 4 (drug acquisition cost)	40	100	0.10	0.10	4	10
Totals	**NA**	**NA**	**1.00**	**1.00**	**71.5**	**77.5**

NA, not applicable.

trees provide a graphic display of treatment options, their outcomes, and the probability of those outcomes occurring.

All decision trees represented graphically usually contain choice and chance nodes. Choice nodes typically depict a point at which a decision needs to be made for the user to progress forward in trying to achieve a desired outcome. Chance nodes have a likely probability of taking place and may or may not be favorable (eg, adverse medication events, additional tests).

- Choice node (box): what follows is under the control of the decision maker.
- Branch: originates from the node; one for each alternative or possible events.
- Chance node (circle): what follows is subject to probabilistic outcome.
- Decision path: sequence of events originating at initial choice node and following a particular course, ending at terminal node (outcome).

Each event in the decision tree can be assigned a probability of occurrence. The sum of the probability values associated with each branch of the tree must equal 1.0 or 100%. See FIGURE 10-1 for a sample decision tree.

The primary literature usually serves as a source for the probabilities, but they can also be derived from consensus panels, experts in the field, and local data. Databases from electronic medical records offer more promising sources for the future, allowing the use of accumulated clinical data or records and outcomes from actual practice to determine predictable scenarios for similar clinical situations. Once probabilities are assigned to all likely discrete events, the sum probabilities of outcomes must be calculated.

Some disease states such as infectious processes lend themselves to defined clinical end points, such a clinical resolution or microbiological cure. Yet some diseases such

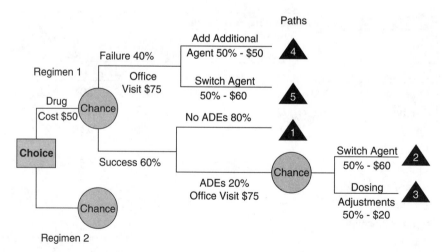

FIGURE 10-1 Sample decision tree.

ADE, adverse drug event.

Table 10-2	Steps Involved in Decision Tree Analysis

1. Define the objectives (state the problem).

2. Identify alternatives to attain desired outcomes.

3. Structure the decision problem as a logical sequence of events (include choice nodes).

4. Characterize known and uncertain events and then establish probabilities of events occurring (include chance nodes).

5. Place values on the resource consumed and calculate expected costs.

6. Perform appropriate calculations.

7. Make a selection based on the results.

8. Conduct a sensitivity analysis (alter various probabilities and/or assumptions to see if the calculated results change).

as hypertension typically use surrogate end points. In the treatment of hypertension, the desired outcome may be a reduction in the incidence of myocardial infarction; however, the surrogate end point assessed is reduced or normalized blood pressure in the patient(s). Utilization of decision trees usually requires several steps, as seen in TABLE 10-2.

An example best illustrates the decision tree process. As seen in Figure 10-1, there is a decision to treat the patient with either regimen 1 or regimen 2. Chance nodes (depicted by circles) and a choice node (depicted by a box) are depicted in this figure as well.

Regimen 1 has the following probabilities: treatment success of 60% and treatment failure of 40%. Associated with treatment success are no adverse drug events (ADEs) 80% of the time and ADEs 20% of the time. ADEs further result in dosing adjustments 50% of the time and switching drugs the other 50%. It is worth noting that even with clinical success, there can be adverse events that are incurred that require additional resources to manage.

Regimen 1 has a treatment failure of 40%, resulting in switching drugs 50% of the time and adding an additional agent the other 50% of the time. Knowing this, the overall probability of an outcome and expected values can be determined and compared with other drug regimens. This step is often referred to as "folding back the decision tree," because to calculate the overall probabilities, you can work from right to left carrying forward each probability.

In regimen 1, the following probabilities can be determined for successful outcomes (60%):

- Path 1: without adverse effects occurs 48% of the time ($0.6 \times 0.8 = 0.48$).
- Path 2: with adverse effects that result in switching to another agent occurs 6% of the time ($0.6 \times 0.2 \times 0.5 = 0.06$).
- Path 3: a successful outcome with adverse effects that results in adjusting the dose of the current agent occurs 6% of the time ($0.6 \times 0.2 \times 0.5 = 0.06$).

Probabilities associated with treatment failures (40% overall) can also be calculated, each being 20% respectively:

- Path 4: failures resulting in switching therapy $(0.40 \times 0.50 = 0.20)$.
- Path 5: failures resulting in additional agents being added $(0.40 \times 0.50 = 0.20)$.

Expected values can then be calculated based on the costs associated with each event in the decision tree. If the occurrence of a successful outcome without adverse effects (path 1) occurs 48% of the time with regimen 1, and the sole costs at this point are related to drug acquisition costs of the agent in this regimen (ie, $50), then the expected value associated with this outcome is $24 $(0.6 \times 0.8 \times \$50 = \$24)$. Likewise, the expected value for a successful outcome with adverse effects that result in switching to another agent (path 2) would be $11.10 based on the following costs: drug acquisition cost of $50, $75 for the second physician office visit due to the adverse event, and $60 for the new agent switched to $[0.6 \times 0.2 \times 0.5 \times (\$50 + \$75 + \$60) = \$11.10]$. In the final scenario for successful outcomes of regimen 1, the expected value for a successful outcome with adverse effects that result in adjusting the dose of the current agent (path 3) would be $8.70 based on the following costs: drug acquisition cost of $50, $75 for the second physician office visit due to the adverse event, and $20 for costs associated with a dosing adjustment $[0.6 \times 0.2 \times 0.5 \times (\$50 + \$75 + \$20) = \$8.70]$. Treatment failure costs would be $37.00 $[0.4 \times 0.5 \times (\$50 + \$75 + \$60) = \$37.00]$ for path 4 and $45.00 $[0.4 \times 0.5 \times (\$50 + \$75 + \$100) = \$45.00]$ for path 5.

Once all expected values are calculated for each possible path in the decision tree, an overall sum of costs associated with the decision tree can be attained. Thus, the overall expected costs for successful outcomes in regimen 1 are $43.80 ($24.10 + $11.10 + $8.70), and the overall treatment failure costs are $82.00 ($37.00 + $45.00). Therefore, the average cost a patient could incur in this model is the sum of $43.80 and $82.00, equaling $125.80. Clearly, the failure paths incur more costs relative to successful outcomes notwithstanding the negative clinical outcomes. These expected values are found in TABLE 10-3.

The same process described earlier would be repeated for regimen 2 and/or other treatments, and the lowest overall expected value would be selected as providing the least overall cost of therapy given the associated successes and failures. For example, if regimen 2 had an overall expected value of $150.00, then regimen 1 would be the preferred agent because its overall expected value is $125.80, or approximately $25 less per patient. It is important to note that these overall expected values are the average cost per patient that could be anticipated because it is not known exactly which patients would be treated with success or failure, and not simply the drug acquisition costs of the respective regimens. In essence, the practitioner does not know when initiating therapy which patient will incur less optimal outcomes and thus more costs related to therapy. Although this $25 difference may not seem like a lot, it certainly adds up when taking care of 10,000 patient lives (resulting in $250,000) or 100,000 patient lives

Table 10-3	Expected Values Associated with the Decision Tree Analysis		
Path	Probabilities	Costs	Expected Values
Regimen 1			
Successful paths			
Path 1	$0.6 \times 0.8 = 0.48$	$50	$24.00
Path 2	$0.6 \times 0.2 \times 0.5 = 0.06$	$50 + $75 + $60	$11.10
Path 3	$0.6 \times 0.2 \times 0.5 = 0.06$	$50 + $75 + $20	$8.70
Subtotals	0.60		$43.80
Failure paths			
Path 4	$0.40 \times 0.50 = 0.20$	$50 + $75 + $60	$37.00
Path 5	$0.40 \times 0.50 = 0.20$	$50 + $75 + $100	$45.00
Subtotals	0.40		$82.00
Total sum	**1.00**		**$125.80**

($2.5 million). Hence, these large dollar amounts from decision analyses get the interest of health care plans and government payers.

As seen in FIGURE 10-2, there is a decision to treat the patient with either medication A or medication B for dyslipidemia (high cholesterol) for secondary prevention of a

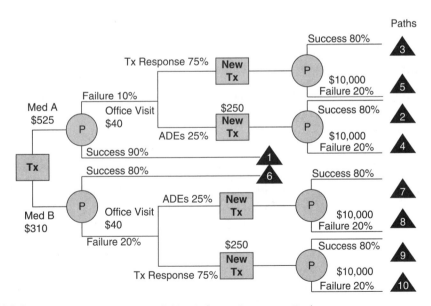

FIGURE 10-2 Simple decision tree for dyslipidemia (secondary prevention).

ADE, adverse drug event; Med, medication; P, probability; Tx, treatment.

Table 10-4	Product Comparison to Treat High Cholesterol
Medication A	Medication B
Higher efficacy (significant LDL reductions)	Lower efficacy (minimal LDL reductions)
Equal safety profile	Equal safety profile
Higher drug cost ($526)	Lower drug cost ($310)
Same dosing regimen (once daily)	Same dosing regimen (once daily)

LDL, low-density lipoprotein.

cardiac event. If patients do not meet success, they incur an office visit for $40 followed by a change in therapy of $250. At this stage of the decisions tree, it is assumed that if patients do not meet with success, they will go on to experience a cardiac event (assuming this requires hospitalization for $10,000). Medication A, which costs $525, has a treatment success of 90% and treatment failure of 10%. Medication B, which costs $310, has a treatment success of 80% and treatment failure of 20%. Specific properties of the medications are provided in TABLE 10-4.

Overall, the probability of success with medication A is 98%, whereas it is 96% with medication B. Based on the decision tree analysis, medication A appears to be the favored agent because the total expected cost is $754.05 versus a total cost of $768.00 for medication B. In addition, medication A is preferred because the cost-effectiveness ratio is more favorable (ie, lower) (TABLE 10-5). The cost-effectiveness ratio can be calculated by dividing the expected value by the overall probability of success for each agent. For each medication, the cost-effectiveness ratios are:

Medication A: $754.05/0.98 = $769.44
Medication B: $768.00/0.96 = $800.00

Thus, the 2% difference in success has an impact on the overall costs of therapy. Again, the total expected value of an agent can be thought of as the average cost to treat a patient because it is not known at the initiation of therapy which patients will encounter success or treatment failure. Or another way to look at this is that if a health plan had 1000 patients to treat, the total expected costs would be as follows:

Medication A: $754.05 × 1000 patients = $754,050
Medication B: $768.00 × 1000 patients = $768,000
                            Variance of $13,950

Health care providers must have the ability to critically review and evaluate decision analysis and the pharmacoeconomic literature as it pertains to their practice. They must be able to determine whether economic evaluations use appropriate methods and have valid results and conclusions and if such results are applicable to their practice environment(s). Drug acquisition costs alone should not be the only factor considered when selecting medication therapies for either individual patients or populations of

Table 10-5	Expected Values Associated with the Decision Tree Analysis		
Path	Probabilities	Costs	Expected Values
Medication A			
Successful paths			
Path 1	0.9 = 0.90	$525	$472.50
Path 2	0.1 × 0.25 × 0.8 = 0.020	$525 + $40 + $250	$16.30
Path 3	0.1 × 0.75 × 0.8 = 0.060	$525 + $40 + $250	$48.90
Subtotals	**0.980**		**$537.70**
Failure paths			
Path 4	0.10 × 0.25 × 0.20 = 0.005	$525 + $40 + $250 + $10,000	$54.10
Path 5	0.10 × 0.75 × 0.20 = 0.015	$525 + $40 + $250 + $10,000	$162.25
Subtotals	**0.02**		**$216.35**
Total sum	**1.00**		$754.05
Cost-effectiveness ratio: $754.05/0.98 = $769.44			
Medication B			
Successful paths			
Path 6	0.8 = 0.80	$310	$248.00
Path 7	0.2 × 0.25 × 0.8 = 0.040	$310 + $40 + $250	$24.00
Path 9	0.2 × 0.75 × 0.8 = 0.120	$310 + $40 + $250	$72.00
Subtotals	**0.960**		**$344.00**
Failure paths			
Path 8	0.20 × 0.25 × 0.20 = 0.010	$310 + $40 + $250 + $10,000	$106.00
Path 10	0.20 × 0.75 × 0.20 = 0.030	$310 + $40 + $250 + $10,000	$318.00
Subtotals	**0.040**		**$424.00**
Total sum	**1.00**		$768.00
Cost-effectiveness ratio: $768.00/0.96 = $800.00			

patients. The full economic impact and clinical outcomes of pharmacotherapeutic-based interventions must not only be determined but be based on probability and be defensible and transparent.

■ References

1. Swalm RO. Utility theory: insights into risk taking. *Harvard Business Review* 1966;44:123–136.
2. Aldag RJ, Stearns TM. Decision-making tools for managing. In: *Cases, Readings, and Special Topics in Management*. Cincinnati, OH: South-Western Publishing Company; 1987:195–225.

Introduction to Economic Analysis, Cost Determinants, and Modeling

Jaewhan Kim, PhD
Junhua Yu, PhD

Learning Objectives

- Describe what economic analysis means.
- Describe why economic evaluation in pharmacoeconomics is important.
- List types of economic analysis.
- List and discuss elements of economic analysis.
- Identify types of costs and discuss how costs can be determined.
- Discuss limitations of economic analysis.

■ Introduction

Under the pressure of increasing costs of health care, as well as concerns over quality and effectiveness, economic analysis has been used by health care policy makers as a decision tool to compare costs with outcomes (ie, economic, clinical, and humanistic outcomes) of interest. In economic evaluations in drug treatment, pharmacoeconomics has been used as another term to indicate such economic evaluations. Given the increasing costs of new medications and the greater emphasis on health care cost containment, pharmacoeconomics plays an important role in the evaluation of drug products and the decision-making process regarding drug coverage policies.

Pharmacoeconomics is a tool used to identify, measure, and compare the costs and outcomes of the use of pharmaceutical products and services. Pharmacoeconomics puts the total cost of drug therapy into relation with the outcomes of the therapy. In pharmacoeconomics, economic evaluations have been popularly used to make decisions in many situations such as development decisions, formulary decisions, and pricing decisions. Making decisions is not limited to pharmacoeconomics because of resource scarcity, which necessitates that choice among alternatives must be made in all areas of human activity. To make better decisions, economic analysis provides important information on how to allocate scare resource efficiently to decision makers.

Economic analysis in pharmacoeconomics identifies and compares the costs and outcomes (ie, economic, clinical, and humanistic outcomes) of pharmaceutical products and services. Tools for examining the impact of alternative drug therapies and other medical interventions and, therefore, providing important information to decision makers are used in pharmacoeconomics.

This chapter describes what types of economic analysis are available, followed by a description of the elements of economic analysis, including types of outcomes, types of costs, and how costs can be determined. However, economic analyses are not perfect models for decision makers, so limitations of economic analysis will also be discussed.

■ Types of Economic Analysis

In economic analysis, to inform decisions between competing therapies, 4 types of economic assessments have been used: cost-minimization analysis (CMA), cost-benefit analysis (CBA), cost-effectiveness analysis (CEA), and cost-utility analysis (CUA) (TABLE 11-1). In all analyses, the commonly necessary factor is cost. In all 4 models, cost is measured by the same way in terms of monetary unit (eg, dollars). However, outcomes in the analyses are determined by different measures. The choice of which type is appropriate is dependent on the study question, the disease or disease state of interest, and the availability of outcome data.

CMA is the simplest form of economic analysis and compares the costs of 2 or more alternatives or treatments. The necessary information is regarding costs without values in outcomes because the outcomes of the interventions under comparison are assumed to be identical or similar. Thus, costs are the only consideration in CMA, so results are expressed in monetary units (eg, dollars). CMA is used to identify the least expensive alternative. CMA can be used to compare brand and generic versions of the same product. Because clinical effects between both products are identical, comparing their costs is fairly simple. After comparison in costs between products, the lower cost agent is selected. CMA can also be used to compare different products. However, as

Table 11-1	Types of Economic Analysis	
Type of Analysis	Costs	Outcomes
Cost-minimization	Monetary units (eg, dollars)	Assumed to be equivalent
Cost-effectiveness	Monetary units (eg, dollars)	Natural units (eg, life-years saved)
Cost-benefit	Monetary units (eg, dollars)	Monetary units (eg, dollars)
Cost-utility	Monetary units (eg, dollars)	Quality-adjusted life-years

soon as there is a difference in the outcomes, CMA is not permitted. Furthermore, CMA is too simple to reflect complex reality, especially in health care.

To account for different outcomes, more complex analyses than CMA have been developed, such as CEA, CBA, and CUA. CEA measures costs in monetary units and effectiveness as outcomes in natural health units such as life-years saved or change in blood pressure. Because costs and effectiveness are measured in noncomparable units (monetary units in costs vs natural units in outcomes), CEA assesses treatment options through use of the incremental cost-effectiveness ratio (ICER) as costs per effectiveness. The ICER is estimated as the incremental difference in cost (cost of drug A vs cost of drug B) between 2 alternatives divided by the incremental difference in effectiveness (effectiveness of drug A vs effectiveness of drug B) between the 2 alternatives.

CBA is similar to CEA in that both assess costs and outcomes of comparative treatments. However, unlike CEA, CBA involves measuring both costs and benefits as outcomes of treatments in monetary terms. By valuing all costs and benefits in the same units (ie, monetary units), CBA compares diverse interventions using the net benefit criterion (ie, benefits minus costs). Because outcomes are measured in monetary units, CBA allows decision makers to compare programs that have different outcomes measures unlike CEA.

CUA is similar to CEA but measures a treatment's effect using the quality of health gained from the treatment (ie, a utility). A common approach to measure health utility is quality-adjusted life-years (QALYs). Then, the results of CUA are described in the additional costs of the treatment with a new drug per unit of health gain measured as QALYs (ie, cost per QALY). There are a number of useful instruments for assessing health-related quality of life such as the Short Form-36, EQ-5D, Health Utility Index, and Quality of Well-Being Scale, which are generic instruments. In addition, disease-specific instruments to measure illness and medical conditions have been developed. For example, the Asthma Quality of Life Questionnaire and Diabetes Quality of Life Questionnaire are designed to measure asthma and diabetes, respectively.

■ Elements of Economic Analysis

To conduct economic analysis, there are 5 essential points: perspective of the analysis, costs, outcomes, discounting costs and outcomes, and addressing uncertainty.

Perspective

Perspective refers to who the target audience is for the economic analysis study. Costs and outcomes to be included in the study are determined from whose perspective the analysis is conducted. Each health care stakeholder possesses different needs and preferences when making decisions on therapies. Therefore, the perspective of the analysis should be determined before conducting the analysis because different points of the perspective influence costs and outcomes differently. What is important to one group may not be relevant to another group. Four categories of perspectives based on health care stakeholders are usually considered: society, the patient, the provider, and the payer. A societal perspective is the broadest perspective and incorporates most costs and outcomes.

The patient or individual perspective incorporates only those costs that are relevant to an individual use of one of the comparators. The provider perspective would incorporate only costs of resources paid for by the hospital/institution. The payer perspective refers to a group or organization that provides payment for health care services to a group or individual. An evaluation using the third-party payer perspective would include the costs of reimbursement to eligible users, but would not include the cost of wages lost by an individual due to an unexpected adverse event from the treatment.

Cost Determinants

Different perspectives exist regarding which costs should be included in an analysis. The cost determination of a therapy contains 3 unique tasks: cost identification, measurement, and valuation. Cost identification indicates that all relevant resources consumed by an intervention relevant to the study perspective should be identified, depending on the perspective of the study. All relevant resources can be directly and indirectly related to a therapy or an intervention. The identification of various types of costs is similar across economic analysis. Measurement refers to the magnitude of resource consumption, which should be quantified. When all relevant resources have been identified, a unit of consumption should be considered.

Valuation refers to conversion of the quantified resources used in the intervention into a monetary value. However, there are different types of costs from different sources. For cost identification, understanding main categories of costs is essential. Costs are derived from multiple sources such as tangible costs and intangible costs.

Tangible costs consist of direct costs and indirect costs. Direct costs include the materials that are directly associated with providing the medical intervention such as drug treatment, hospital facilities, and personnel and laboratory costs. Indirect costs include items such as lost wages, lost time from work, and costs associated with traveling for physicians' office visits. Intangible costs represent unquantifiable costs such as the value of improved health after treatment, pain, or suffering. However, it is difficult to place a monetary value on and thus measure intangible costs. These costs have been measured and valued through the willingness-to-pay approach in CBA.

Measuring Outcomes

Three main approaches exist to measuring outcomes: clinical end points, quality-of-life measures, and willingness to pay. Clinical end points, such as reduction in the number of strokes, reduced mortality, and increased years of life, have been used as outcomes in CEA. Utility-based quality-of-life measures have been used as outcomes in CUA. The benefits of an intervention in CBA are measured as the willingness to pay of the individuals who benefit from the intervention.

Discounting Cost and Outcomes

The costs and outcomes associated with interventions may be incurred at different points in time. However, most cases may have different timing of costs and outcomes. For comparison between interventions in economic analysis, costs and outcomes must be converted to have same time profile by adjusting values in costs and outcomes. Discounting is a basic principle of economics that the value of a dollar today is worth more than the value of a dollar in the future. Discounting allows the future costs to be brought to the current time so that these values can be compared fairly. However, there is no consensus as to which discount rate to use; instead, a range of 3% to 5% is common.

Sensitivity Analysis for Uncertainty and Variability

The uncertainty due to lack of precision in estimations, variability of results in the published literature, or methodologic issues based on distributional assumptions should be addressed in the economic analysis. One approach to address the uncertainty is a sensitivity analysis. A sensitivity analysis tests all the assumptions used in the model and enables the impact of "best-case" and "worst-case" scenarios on the baseline findings to be investigated.

Three methods of sensitivity analyses are commonly used: one-way sensitivity analysis, multi-way sensitivity analysis, and probabilistic sensitivity analysis. One-way sensitivity analysis has been used to consider a single parameter in the model, holding other parameters constant. Multi-way sensitivity analysis refers to changing multiple parameters in the model and reporting changes in results. Probabilistic sensitivity analysis is another method to measure uncertainty and variability by applying values taken from diverse probability distributions over parameters of interest. Using one form of sensitivity analysis in economic analysis is required.

■ Modeling in Economic Evaluations

In economic analysis, sources of costs and outcomes on the treatments are derived from literature, national and commercial data sets, and expert opinion. However, time restraints and incomplete data sets constrain researchers conducting economic analysis. Under such limitations in economic analysis, modeling is an analytical tool that has been used to construct hypothetical situations. The most commonly used models in economic assessment of treatments is decision analysis.

Decision analysis is a systematic approach to decision making under uncertainty. With this technique, researchers are able to compare alternative management or treatment strategies to provide an informed way to choose between the options. Modeling techniques associated with decision analysis allow options to be quantified and to enter directly into the decision process. Consequences can include anything from symptom reduction to adverse events, whereas costs can encompass both monetary and nonmonetary costs associated directly or indirectly with the intervention. This modeling allows for the inclusion of uncertainty, which is an important component of real-world clinical treatment.

Uncertainty enters into clinical treatment through many avenues, including whether an intervention will have its desired effect and whether a patient will develop complications. The goal of a decision model is to help a decision maker understand the trade-off between the risks and the benefits of several alternatives. Therefore, a prerequisite for performing a decision analysis is uncertainty regarding the best alternative.

There are 2 main types of decision models: decision trees and Markov models. For decision analysis, which considers the average patient experience, the decision tree and the Markov model are the most often used forms of cohort model in decision analysis. However, they are not mutually exclusive methods in decision analysis. Therefore, they can be used together for a decision model.

A decision tree is a way to graphically represent the sequence of events (treatments and disease states) and is the simplest form of decision analysis. The decision tree is a commonly used method in decision analyses. Although appealing because of its visual simplicity, this technique has several limitations. The first is that decision trees can become quite "bushy." Many diseases and associated treatment options are fairly complex, so trying to depict every relevant branch makes the model unwieldy. A second related limitation is that decision trees allow movement to occur in only one direction. It is difficult to depict transitions back and forth between disease states without running into the bushy tree problem. Finally, the processes that are reflected in the tree are essentially static. In other words, there is no way to make the model dynamic by incorporating events that take place over time. This lack of time dimension in decision trees makes it impossible to discount outcomes.

Markov models are another type of decision model and are able to overcome the limitations of decision trees. Markov models are able to incorporate complexities of disease states in a much more manageable fashion, because they are recursive, meaning that they allow for transitions back and forth between disease states over time. In addition, their construction allows for events over time to be explicitly modeled. As a result, Markov models have been used to study the progression of many chronic diseases. Another advantage of these models is the ability to assign value to time spent in each health state.

One of the representative methods for solving a Markov model is called a Monte Carlo simulation. In this technique, the values of the inputs to the Markov model are taken to be random draws from a distribution of probabilities. Although they overcome many of the shortcomings of decision trees, Markov models are also not without limitations. The biggest problem with Markov models is that transition probabilities from one health state to another are only determined by the current state and not by previous ones. For this reason, it is sometimes said that Markov models are "memory-less."

◾ Limitations of Economic Analysis

Economic analyses are useful tools to assess therapies or interventions. Although the analyses are useful, individual analysis should be conducted carefully, because there are several limitations of economic analysis. First, economic analyses do not usually incorporate the importance of the distribution of costs and outcomes among different patient or population groups into the analysis. Second, the various forms of analysis embody different equity criteria. Third, economic analyses assume that resources freed or saved by preferred interventions will not in fact be wasted but will be employed in alternative worthwhile interventions. Lastly, economic analyses are themselves a costly activity.

However, under the pressure of increasing costs in health care as well as concerns over quality and effectiveness, economic analysis has become an attractive decision tool for health care policy makers to compare costs with outcomes, given finite resources.

◾ Additional Resources

Bala MV, Mauskipf JA, Wood LL. Willingness to pay as a measure of health benefits. *Pharmacoeconomics.* 1999;15:9–18.

Bambha K, Kim WR. Cost-effectiveness analysis and incremental cost-effectiveness ratios: uses and pitfalls. *Eur J Gastroenterol Hepatol.* 2004;16:519–526.

Basskin L. *Practical Pharmacoeconomics: How to Design, Perform and Analyze Outcomes Research.* Cleveland, OH: Advanstar Communications, Inc.; 1998.

Bootman JL, Townsend RJ, McGhan WF. *Principles of Pharmacoeconomics.* Cincinnati, OH: Harvey Whitney Books Company; 2005.

Briggs A. Statistical approaches to handing uncertainty in health economic evaluation. *Eur J Gastroenterol Hepatol.* 2004;16:551–561.

Briggs A, Sculpher M, Claxton K. *Decision Modelling for Health Economic Evaluation.* New York, NY: Oxford University Press; 2005.

Chumney E, Simpson K. *Methods and Designs for Outcomes Research.* Bethesda, MD: American Society of Health-System Pharmacists, Inc.; 2006.

Deverill M, Brazier J, Green C, Booth A. The use of QALY and non-QALY measures of health-related quality of life. *Pharmacoeconomics.* 1998;13:411–420.

Drummond MF, Sculpher MJ, Torrance GW, et al. *Methods for the Economic Evaluation of Health Care Programmes.* New York, NY: Oxford University Press; 2005.

Johannesson M, Jönsson B, Karlsson G. Outcome measurement in economic evaluation. *Health Econ.* 1996;5:279–296.

Johnson N, Nash D. *The Role of Pharmacoeconomics in Outcomes Management.* Belcamp, MD: American Hospital Publishing, Inc.; 1996.

Kim J, Nelson R, Biskupiak J. Decision analysis: a primer and application to pain-related studies. *J Pain Palliat Care Pharmacother.* 2008;22:192–299.

Liljas B. How to calculate indirect costs in economic evalutions. *Pharmacoeconomics.* 1998;13:1–7.

Moayyedi P, Mason J. Cost-utility and cost-benefit analysis: how did we get here and where are we going? *Eur J Gastroenterol Hepatol.* 2004;16:527–534.

Pizzi L, Lofland J. *Economic Evaluation in US Health Care: Principles and Applications.* Sudbury, MA: Jones and Bartlett Publishers, Inc.; 2006.

Cost-of-Illness Analysis and Budget Impact Models

Steven E. Marx, PharmD, RPh

Learning Objectives

- Differentiate between the different types of costs used to portray a disease, and describe how the perspectives may influence the costs used in the analysis.

- Identify potential sources for defining costs in a cost-of-illness study, and describe the complexities associated with describing costs.

- Define costs from a disease state perspective and the importance of understanding the patient characteristics in order to translate them in the desired population.

- Define and discuss the importance of discounting when utilizing and assessing costs over multiple years.

- Describe the format for developing a budget impact model and describe how to interpret the results.

- Identify costs related to drug treatment that are appropriate for the perspective chosen to describe the budget impact over time.

- Discuss the uses and limitations of using a budget impact model for comparing drugs for formulary inclusion.

■ Introduction

Health economic analysis always requires a researcher to define the cost of care. Although it may seem to be the simplest task, it typically proves to be the most difficult. Similar to purchasing car, the actual cost is difficult to define. There is the sticker price, the dealership price, the price you pay, and the price others pay. To further complicate the final cost, there is also the price for your trade in, cash back, and lower interest rates. On top of all that, there can be destination charges, taxes, and title and license fees. Similarly, health care costs can be just as complex. The term *costs* implies what someone pays for a product, but this may not always be the case.

Typically there are 3 types of costs: direct, indirect, and tangible costs. Direct costs are those costs directly related to the disease in question. Examples of direct costs of hypertension could include nutritional support to reduce salt intake, medications for the treatment of high blood pressure, physician office visits, emergency room visits for hypertensive-related admissions, hospitalizations associated with hypertension, and exercise/health club memberships to reduce weight. Indirect costs of hypertension include spouse or family member time off from work to go with the individual to office visits.

Depending on the perspective of the analysis, the costs will change. For example, for a prescription for hypertension medication, the patient's costs include the co-pay and a portion of their health insurance costs, whereas the pharmacist's costs include the cost of the medication and personnel costs, and the health insurer's costs include the amount reimbursed to the pharmacist. Therefore, when evaluating a cost study, the first question that needs to be answered is whose perspective is the analysis assessing.

In health care, costs are further categorized by acquisition costs for product or service; amount charged to the provider, patient, or insurance carrier; or the reimbursement to the provider or institution. Acquisition costs are typically what a patient, provider, institution, or pharmacist pays for the product. For medications, the acquisition costs may be defined as the invoice price, direct purchase price, average wholesale price, or average selling price. The invoice price may or may not be the true acquisition cost, if a rebate or discount is not included on the invoice. Direct purchase price is typically lower than purchasing a product through a wholesaler; however, there is typically a minimum quantity required and a long time between the date order and the date received. Purchasing an item through a wholesaler is slightly more expensive than buying direct; however, the item is usually obtained within 24 hours. The amount charged typically covers the cost of the product and/or service plus some mark up. For outpatient prescriptions, there is usually a dispensing fee added to each prescription dispensed. Reimbursement is what is received from the insurer for services rendered. In most cases, what is charged in health care is higher than what is reimbursed, because often third-party contracts through insurance companies have discounted rates over the typical and customary charges.

There are many sources to find prescription costs. The *Red Book* provides medication direct prices and average wholesale prices (AWP)[1]. Average wholesale price refers to the average price at which a wholesaler sells medications to physicians and pharmacists. It is not defined in law or regulation and does not account for any discounts. In contrast, the average sales price factors in discounts and rebates. Medicare reimbursement for medications, physician office visits, laboratory tests, and hospitalizations is available through the Resource-Based Relative Value Scale (RBRVS)[2].

Some state-specific reimbursements are available using Internet searches. The *DRG Handbook* provides average institutional costs, charges, and reimbursements for hospitalizations, including a breakdown of costs by services, states, and types of hospitals.[3] National, regional, and state estimates of hospital use and costs by payer are also available through the Internet for United States.[4] Although this source is free, the latest data are at least 2 years old. Some state medicaid databases are available for research purposes through the state. The California Medicaid database is one of the largest. Other commercial insurance databases are available for purchase. There are 31 US databases listed on the International Society for Pharmacoeconomics and Outcomes Research (ISPOR) Web site and 92 international databases.[5] Although US databases are typically very robust, non-US databases are much more limited.

Other potential sources include disease-specific registries. The US Renal Database Service (USRDS) is one example of a disease state database.[6] The USRDS is a national data system that collects, analyzes, and distributes information about end-stage renal disease (ESRD) in the United States. This database explores characteristics of the ESRD population, prevalence and incidence of ESRD, and trends in mortality and disease rates and investigates relationships among patient demographics, treatment modalities, and morbidity. Additionally, this source explores the predialysis databases such as the National Health and Nutrition Examination Survey (NHANES)[7], Medstat Market Scan,[8] Ingenix i3,[9] and Medicare[10] databases.

■ Cost of Illness

Cost-of-illness studies describe the total health care costs associated with a specific disease. How the study defines the health state is critical in representing the disease. Although International Classification of Diseases (ICD-9)[11] codes are usually used to define a disease state, these codes may not always be available within the data set or specific enough to describe the disease in question. Occasionally, surrogate measures are used, such as medications. For example, 2 prescriptions for insulin may be used for type 1 diabetes. The purpose of 2 prescriptions is to eliminate the possibility of a coding error.

When defining costs associated with a disease state, costs are broken down into at least 3 types of services: prescriptions, outpatient services, and inpatient services. Over-the-counter medications are usually difficult to identify in a database and typically require a prospective approach to collect. Databases that include only specific pharmacies have the potential to miss some medications if a prescription is filled outside of the network. However, insurance claims databases will capture all reimbursed claims, although typically not over-the-counter medications.

However, if a specific medication, such as lifestyle medications (eg, Viagra, Cialis), is not reimbursed, these medications may not be available through an insurance claims database. It is important to realize the limitation of the number of medications if the cost per prescription is calculated. Prescriptions may be filled for different lengths of treatment, thereby confounding the analysis. Disease-specific medication costs can be specified based on American Hospital Formulary Service (AHFS)[12] number or other drug classification codes. Similar limitations are seen with other costs.

Physician office visits in electronic medical record databases are typically limited to general practitioners (eg, internist, family practice, pediatrics), thus missing specialist's costs. For certain disease states, rehabilitation and caregiver costs are included. Rehabilitations costs are important in surgical procedures such as hip or knee replacement, stroke, or amputations. Caregiver costs are important in, for example, Alzheimer disease, dementia, and surgical procedures. However, caregiver costs are limited to caregiver and societal perspectives.

Presenteeism and absenteeism are important in any disease state that interferes with a patient's ability to work and are limited to employer, employee, and societal perspectives. Presenteeism is a patient's work productivity while at work, whereas absenteeism is simply time off from work, both partial days and full days off. Disease states that interfere with a patient's performance, such as allergies, migraine headaches, lower back pain, and arthritis, can affect a patient's presenteeism by having a negative impact on the patient's work productivity, yet may or may not impact the patient's absenteeism. Costs for salaries lost can be found on various Web sites including www. worldsalaries.org.

Another part of human capital is household expense. If a disease impairs a patient's ability to perform household chores and activities of daily living, then these costs are associated with societal perspectives. League tables of household chores by age and sex are available.[13]

Because the use of costs varies within perspectives, it is important for cost-of-illness studies to include health care resource utilizations. Therefore, another perspective could apply the average costs of the resource utilizations to estimate the cost of illness. Because costs are typically right-skewed, with some patients having no costs, specific methodologies must be used to compare costs. The appropriate technique is a generalized linear model using gamma distribution with a log link function to adjust for variables for potential confounders.

The cost of secondary hyperparathyroidism (SHPT) in diabetic patients with chronic kidney disease was recently published in the literature. The study examined the cost and utilization of medications and outpatient and inpatient services compared with diabetics patients with chronic kidney disease without SHPT. In this cost analysis, diabetic patients with chronic kidney disease and SHPT had annual costs per patient of $91,365 ± $290,243, with a mean of 75.6 ± 47.7 annual prescriptions, 121.4 ± 100.1 outpatient annual visits, and 2.6 ± 5.6 hospitalizations per year. Cardiovascular-related hospitalizations were the primary cost driver for this illness. Total health care costs were 320% ($P < 0.0001$) higher in diabetic chronic kidney disease patients with SHPT compared with diabetic chronic kidney disease patients without SHPT.[14]

■ Budget Impact Models

Budget impact models are developed to demonstrate the impact of cost over a period of time for a country, insurance carrier, hospital, or institution. Budget impact models express the increase in costs to drug budgets and any consequences of other budgets, such as hospitalizations or outpatient visits.[15]

Table 12-1	Epidemiology of Hemodialysis Patients with SHPT
Population = 58.057 million	
Population growth per year = 0.1%	
Prevalence of hemodialysis per year = 665 per million	
Incidence of hemodialysis per year = 104 per million	
Mortality of hemodialysis per year = 13.3%	
Percentage of patients with SHPT = 40%	
Percentage of patient eligible for treatment = 100%	

To assess these costs, one must understand the epidemiology of the disease as it relates to medication use (eg, pharmacoepidemiology). The incidence and prevalence of the disease are often included in this analysis to determine the number of patients eligible for treatment. In addition, the drug utilization or uptake is estimated for each year. Therefore, the cost of the present drug is replaced with the cost of the new drug. Although there is no standard duration of time for a budget impact model, a 3- to 5-year time horizon is typically assessed. For example, the incidence and prevalence of SHPT in hemodialysis are well understood in the United States. In 2006, the US incidence of hemodialysis was 360 cases per million lives, and the prevalence of hemodialysis was 1626 cases per million lives. In patients with hemodialysis, approximately 60% receive a vitamin D receptor activator for SHPT.[16] Similar to cost-of-illness studies, a budget impact analysis must define the perspective. For many non-US countries, the perspective is the ministry of health in the respective country.

To estimate the current and future number of patients treated for SHPT in ESRD, one needs to know the estimated patient growth, prevalence of hemodialysis, incidence of hemodialysis, mortality of hemodialysis, percentage of hemodialysis patients with SHPT, and percentage of patients eligible for treatment (TABLE 12-1).

Year 1 number of patients treated for SHPT is calculated using the following formula: population × prevalence of hemodialysis × percentage of patients with SHPT × percentage of patients eligible. Future years are calculated as follows: year $(n - 1)$ × $(1 -$ mortality$)$ + population × $(1 +$ growth$)$ × incidence × percentage of patients with SHPT × percentage eligible (TABLE 12-2).

Table 12-2	Projections for Hemodialysis Patients with SHPT
First-year number of patients treated for SHPT = 15,443: [(58.057 million × 665 per million) × 40% with SHPT] × 100% treated for the disease	
Second-year number of patients treated for SHPT = 15,807: 15,443 patients × $(1 - 13.3\%)$ + $(\{[58.057 × (1 + 0.1\%)] × 104$ per million$\} × 40\%$ with SHPT$)$ × 100% treated for the disease	
Third-year number of patients treated for SHPT = 16,125: 15,807 patients × $(1 - 13.3\%)$ + $\{[58.057$ million × $(1 + 0.1\%)^2 × 104$ per million$] × 40\%$ with SHPT$\}$ × 100% treated for the disease	

For simplicity, the actual model is usually built in Microsoft Excel. The advantage of using this software is familiarity of the software by decision makers and the transparency of the calculations. As part of the calculations, discounting is an important concept when assessing costs. Discounting is a method used to adjust future costs and benefits to their present costs.[17] Typically cost are discounted between 3% and 5% per year using the following formula: $y = x/(1 + r)^n$, where y is the future value, x is the present value, r is the discount rate, and n is the number of years. Simply stated, future costs are higher than present value.

As with any cost analysis, the perspective must first be defined. The perspective will define what cost(s) will be included in the budget impact model. Therefore, a model will need to be versatile if the model will be used for assessing the cost impact for more than one country, institution, or pharmacy benefit manager. Although most models typically only include the cost of the medication, other health care resource utilization may be affected. Some medications may eliminate the need for additional medications, decrease the number of laboratory tests, reduce the number of office visits, or reduce the number of hospitalizations. A model needs to have the flexibility to include or exclude these costs, depending on which costs are important to the decision maker.

For the budget impact model, the yearly medication cost must be calculated for the present treatment A plus the new competing therapy B. For each year, the percentage treated with treatment A and treatment B is estimated. Essentially, the model predicts how much market share treatment will be obtained in the first year. The following example (seen in Tables 12-3 to 12-5) assumes treatment A (a new treatment) costs $2000 per year, and treatment B (the standard of care) costs $1000 per year, and it's predicted that treatment A will demand 20%, 40%, and 60% of the market share in the first, second, and third years when introduced to the market.

The standard-of-care treatment B costs $15,443,000 per year: 15,443 patients × $1,000 per patient per year (TABLE 12-3).

Total cost in the first year equals $18,531,600 ($6,177,200 for treatment A + $12,354,400 for treatment B), increasing the cost of treating this disease in the first year an additional $3,088,600 ($18,531,600 − $15,443,000). In the second year, the number of patients increased to 15,807 patients (TABLE 12-4).

Table 12-3	Budget Impact Model, First Year	
First Year	Treatment A	Treatment B
Number of patients	15,443	15,443
Market share	20%	80%
Cost of treatment per year	$2000	$1000
Total cost	$6,177,200	$12,354,400

Table 12-4	Budget Impact Model, Second Year	
Second Year	Treatment A	Treatment B
Number of patients	15,807	15,807
Market share	40%	60%
Cost of treatment per year	$2000	$1000
Total cost	$12,645,600	$9,484,200

Total cost in the second year equals $22,129,800 ($12,645,600 for treatment A + $9,484,200 for treatment B), increasing the second year costs by $3,598,200 ($22,129,800 − $18,531,600). In the third year, the number of patients increased to 16,125 patients (TABLE 12-5).

Total cost in the third year equals $25,800,000 ($19,350,000 for treatment A + $6,450,000 for treatment B), increasing the third year costs by $3,670,200 ($25,800,000 − $22,129,800).

If additional cost savings can be achieved with treatment A, additional analysis should be performed. Typically, budget impact models are developed for individuals with a financial background and with some type of medical background or experience. Therefore, additional potential cost savings may require additional explanations. The primary purpose of budget impact models is to predict the financial consequences of adding a new drug to the formulary.

■ Summary

Cost-of-illness studies describe the burden and natural history of the disease. The burden is measured as resources and costs. Resources are typically described as medications, outpatient visits and inpatient units, and costs are generally the most difficult to define. Budget impact analysis describes the financial impact for a defined perspective. While it is important to understand the impact on specific budgets, health care decision makers may consider the overall budget impact. Budget impact analysis informs health care decision maker of the estimated future costs of new medications or technology.

Table 12-5	Budget Impact Model, Third Year	
Third Year	Treatment A	Treatment B
Number of patients	16,125	16,125
Market share	60%	40%
Cost of treatment per year	$2000	$1000
Total cost	$19,350,000	$6,450,000

■ References

1. http://www.micromedex.com/products/redbook/awp. Accessed June 11, 2011.
2. http://rbrvs.net. Accessed June 11, 2011.
3. http://www.solucient.com/publications/books/los.shtml. Accessed June 11, 2011.
4. http://hcupnet.ahrq.gov. Accessed June 11, 2011.
5. http://www.ispor.org/DigestOfIntDB/CountryList.aspx. Accessed June 11, 2011.
6. http://www.usrds.org. Accessed June 11, 2011.
7. http://www.cdc.gov/nchs/nhanes.html. Accessed June 11, 2011.
8. http://marketscan.thomsonreuters.com/marketscanportal. Accessed June 11, 2011.
9. http://www.ingenix.com/health-plans/solutions/provider-network-optimization-health. Accessed June 11, 2011.
10. http://www.medicare.gov/Download/DownloadDB.asp. Accessed June 11, 2011.
11. http://www.ama-assn.org/ama/pub/physician-resources/solutions-managing-your-practice/coding-billing-insurance/cpt/announcements-reports/for-ama-icd-9-cm.page. Accessed June 11, 2011.
12. http://www.ahfsdruginformation.com. Accessed June 11, 2011.
13. Haddix AC, Teutsch SM, Corso PS. *Prevention Effectiveness, A Guide to Decision Analysis and Economic Evaluation.* New York: Oxford University Press; 2003.
14. Schumock GT, Andress DL, Marx SE, Sterz R, Joyce AT, Kalantar-Zadeh K. Association of secondary hyperparathyroidism with CKD progression, health care costs and survival in diabetic predialysis CKD patients. *Nephron Clin Pract.* 2009;113(1):c54–61.
15. Mauskopf JA, et al. Principles of Good Practice for Budget Impact Analysis: report of the ISPOR task force on good research practices —budget impact analysis. *Value in Health* 2007;10:336–347.
16. http://www.usrds.org. Accessed June 11, 2011.
17. Berger ML, Bingefors K, Hedblom EC, Pashos CL, Torrance GW. *Health Care Cost, Quality, and Outcomes, ISPOR Book of Terms.* Lawrenceville, NJ: ISPOR; 2003:71.

Cost-Effectiveness Analysis, Cost-Utility Analysis, and Cost-Benefit Analysis

Junhua Yu, PhD
Jaewhan Kim, PhD

Learning Objectives

- Discuss what cost-benefit analysis is and when the analysis is appropriate.
- Describe willingness to pay as an outcome measure in cost-benefit analysis.
- Discuss limitations of cost-benefit analysis.
- Discuss what cost-effectiveness analysis is and when the analysis is appropriate.
- Discuss outcomes in cost-effectiveness analysis and cost-effectiveness ratios.
- Discuss limitations of cost-effectiveness analysis.
- Discuss what cost-utility analysis is and when the analysis is appropriate.
- Describe quality-adjusted life-years as outcomes in cost-utility analysis.
- Discuss limitations of cost-utility analysis.
- Compare and contrast the three cost analysis techniques.

■ Cost-Effectiveness Analysis

Cost-effectiveness analysis (CEA) is the most common type of pharmacoeconomic analysis for evaluation of health intervention programs. It has been widely used across different disease categories and for different types of treatments, such as comparison of radiofrequency ablation with nephron-spring surgery for small unilateral renal cell carcinoma,[1] comparisons of different types of triptans in acute migraine managements,[2] and evaluation of community-based programs aiming to promote healthy lifestyles to prevent type 2 diabetes.[3]

CEA measures costs in dollars and outcomes in natural units that may vary across disease states. The choice of particular outcomes measures is usually dictated by the disease states. A CEA study comparing the cost effectiveness of prophylactic medications used the percentage reduction in monthly frequency of headache as the outcome measures.[4] In an effort to estimate the cost effectives of an inhaled corticosteroid/long-acting β_2-adrenoceptor agonist (β_2-agonist) combination in treating chronic obstructive pulmonary disease, Spencer et al[5] focused on the outcomes of the risk of exacerbations and mortality. In the context of the health care interventions targeted at cardiovascular diseases, the incidence of acute coronary syndrome (hospitalized angina, acute myocardial infarction) or stroke was considered as the outcome of a hypothetical cardiovascular preventive program.[6] The primary reasons for those outcomes adopted in those studies are that they are routinely measured in clinical trials and are familiar to physicians or other practitioners.

The advantage associated with using a specific health outcome is that it offers easy interpretation and immediate application by practitioners. One can also easily see that a disadvantage of CEA is that it cannot provide valid comparison among alternatives that used different clinical units. For example, it does not make sense to conduct CEA to compare the outcomes of antihypertensive drugs (which may be measured as mm Hg change in blood pressure to determine the efficacy in a clinical trial) with the outcomes of antidiabetic drugs (which may be measured by reductions in hemoglobin A1c). In addition, even if products for the same disease are compared, it is not necessarily the case that only one single clinical end point is important. For example, when measuring the efficacy of 6 types of triptans in treating acute migraine, Kelman and Von Seggern[7] looked at multiple outcome measures: (1) pain free at 2 hours after dosing; (2) no recurrence; (3) no rescue headache medication use for 2 to 24 hours; and (4) no adverse events.

Methods

Identify the Alternatives to be Evaluated

The first step in conducting a CEA is to clearly identify the treatment interventions or programs to be evaluated. It is worthwhile to spend some time clarifying the targeted population in terms of age, disease categories, and stage of the disease, and the prevailing competitive intervention or programs relevant to the alternatives being evaluated. It is also important to define the decision makers to whom the message of the study will be relevant.

Collect Data to Identify the Costs

It is crucial to collect high-quality data about cost associated with the treatment and management of the disease from various resources. If the study is conducted from the perspective of society (often considered another separate step), direct costs and indirect costs are also recommended to be estimated. Direct costs might include the treatment procedure and medicines, which can usually be identified in randomized controlled trials or secondary resources such as physicians' fees, the *Red Book*, or the literature of studies of economic burden for that disease. For example, in a study by Brown et al,[4] the costs incurred to a migraine patient using prophylactic medications include physician visits, hospitalization, emergency room visits, acute medications, and daily prophylactic medicine.

In addition to direct costs, CEA often incorporates indirect costs as a result of disease from the society's or employer's perspective. However, there are no universally accepted standards for measurement of indirect costs. The predominate approach seen in the existing literature is the human capital method, which is based on the economic theory that the time patients lose because of a medical condition or its treatment can be translated into forgone wages by attaching a value corresponding to patients' hourly wage rate to the amount of time lost.[8] However, this approach has been subject to considerable debate and criticism[9] primarily because it tends to overestimate the real productivity loss by overlooking the fact that patients might manage to make up the work by themselves or shifting work hours with others.

Collect Data to Identify the Effectiveness

The major sources of data on effectiveness seen in recent studies have been the existing medical literature for clinical trials. Sometimes the published meta-analysis studies can serve as an excellent source of data on effectiveness. Although it has been a common practice to conduct CEA along with clinical trial studies, there is some criticism for this approach. The primary concern stems from the differences between the highly controlled experimental environment in randomized controlled trials (RCTs) and the real-world practice. Because of the controlled conditions in RCTs, such as homogeneous patients, close surveillance, and high adherence with medications that tend to augment the benefit of the medications, it is doubted that the effectiveness measured in RCTs remains the same as that observed in actual clinical use, where all of the conditions beneficial for the performance of interventions in RCTs no longer apply.

However, the existing source of RCT data is easily accessible for economic analysts primarily because of the series of phase trials required by regulatory approval of pharmaceuticals. Therefore, researchers often find themselves in a dilemma of transforming the less than ideal data into useful information for decision makers. Some limitations associated with using RCT data can be accounted for by advanced methodologies, which we will explain later in the section on sensitivity analysis. Another way to overcome the shortfalls is via epidemiologic modeling, which involves the integration of data from clinical trials with those from alternative sources such as retrospective studies based on electronic medical records, pharmacy claims data, and patient surveys that attempt to further verify and validate the RCT outcomes. It is expected that this will allow for evaluation of the broader and longer term impact of interventions.

Design the Model

The model used in CEA can be considered as a mathematical relationship between all the input (eg, specific health care utilization, price for each unit of item of resource, and natural evolution of the disease across different stages) and the output (total cost and health outcomes for each alternative being evaluated) of the CEA study. A model should be specific enough to reflect the natural history of the disease and the various impacts of the interventions on the progress of the disease while avoiding unnecessary details that can damage its generalizability and applicability. There are 2 types of models widely used in the existing CEA literature: decision tree and Markov models. The choice of the type of model is often determined by the nature of disease that the intervention is targeted for and the availability of the data. It has been argued that the Markov model has a unique advantage in simulating the progress of diseases that have relapse patterns or a long monitoring period, which would entail an overwhelming complicated tree format in decision tree models.[10] For example, Bodger et al[11] used a Markov model to represent the natural course of Crohn disease for a duration of 60 years to assist estimation of lifetime costs and effectiveness of infliximab and adalimumab in adult patients. Sher et al[12] developed a Markov model to describe how breast cancer evolves among different disease states, including local recurrence, distant recurrence, recovery after salvage mastectomy, and distant metastasis in the 15 year follow-up after radiotherapy for early-stage breast cancer.

Results of the Base Case Analysis

There are various ways to report the results of CEA. Apart from total cost and effectiveness associated with the alternatives, another measure that is sometimes reported in CEA is the average cost-effectiveness ratio (CER) for each alternative. The CER is calculated by dividing the total cost incurred for achieving a certain amount of units of clinical benefit by that number of units. However, this information will be useful only when the decision makers have the option of leaving the patients untreated and intend to make the comparison of the intervention versus no intervention. Unfortunately, these sorts of comparisons are less likely to be of relevance in the real world because they assume that leaving the patient untreated is an option if the treatment is too expensive. More often, the decision is to whether we should choose this treatment versus another treatment in order to maximize the improvement in health outcomes.

To answer these types of questions, an incremental cost-effectiveness ratio (ICER) is often calculated. The ICER is the ratio of the difference in costs divided by the difference in outcomes. The mathematical formula is as follows:

$$ICER = \frac{\text{Cost of the new treatment} - \text{Cost of the base treatment}}{\text{Effect of the new treatment} - \text{Effect of the base treatment}}$$

As a result, there are 4 possible outcomes associated with this calculation as shown in the cost-effectiveness plane in FIGURE 13-1.

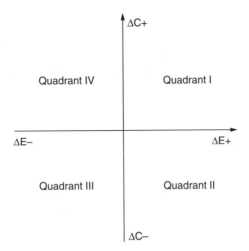

FIGURE 13-1 Incremental cost-effectiveness plane.

When the ICER is positive, the comparison can be either in quadrant I or III.

A. If the new alternative is both more expensive and more effective, the ratio will fall into quadrant I. Of course, a lower ICER will be preferred in this case. A higher ICER will require decision makers to have higher willingness to pay in order for the new technology to be chosen as the favored strategy.

B. If the new alternative costs less but offers less health benefits, the ratio will fall into quadrant III. This is the situation where decision maker will answer the question of whether the lower price of the new treatment technology is justified by the lower cost.

When the ICER is negative, the comparison can be either in quadrant II or quadrant IV.

C. If the new alternative is more costly but less effective (quadrant IV), then the new technology is dominated.

D. If the new alternative costs less and is more effective (quadrant II), then the new technology will be referred as a dominant strategy; that is, it is cost effective regardless of the level of willingness to pay by decision makers.

Consider an example of how to calculate ICER. In a CEA, Buti et al[13] first identified tenofovir to be the most efficacious treatment in terms of the highest number of life-years saved in treating chronic hepatitis B, compared with all of the other therapeutic agents (ie, lamivudine, adefovir, telbivudine, entecavir) approved for this condition in Europe. Because this strategy (ie, tenofovir) dominates all of the other agents except for lamivudine (ie, lower costs and higher number of life-years gained), the ICER for only tenofovir was calculated using lamivudine as the reference alternative, which was $9168 less per life-year as compared with lamivudine. The incremental cost of using tenofovir rather than lamivudine is $172,734 − $1,624,015, whereas the difference in life-years saved between the 2 agents is 19.28 − 17.44; thus, ICER is calculated as: ($172,734 − $1,624,015)/(19.28 − 17.44) = $1,451,281/1.84 = 788,740.

One can quickly see that the using ICER alone in presenting the results can be ambiguous. For example, a relatively small positive ICER can be driven either by a small numerator (a small increase in cost) or a large denominator (a large gain in effectiveness). In addition, a negative ICER can represent 2 dramatically different scenarios: the new technology being either a dominant strategy or a dominated strategy. Moreover, ICER is an appropriate measure only when no dominance exists. So the ICER itself conveys limited information to decision makers. Finally, it is worth mentioning that the ratio does not have a linear property, which would pose a problem for statistical inferences once uncertainty about the cost and effectiveness measures are introduced.

In addition to ICER, another technique, referred to as the incremental net benefit (INB),[14] has been suggested to overcome the aforementioned limitation of ICER. The estimate of INB involves setting the value of maximum acceptable willingness to pay (WTP). INB is calculated by the following equation:

$$INB = WTP \times [(\text{Effect of the new treatment} - \text{Effect of the base treat}) - (\text{Cost of the new treatment} - \text{Cost of the base treatment})]$$

There are 2 advantages of INB compared to ICER. First, INB has straightforward implications. A positive INB implies that the new intervention is deemed cost effective given a certain level of WTP because the extra benefit outweighs the extra costs. Conversely, a negative INB implies that society does not consider the extra benefit worth the increased cost. In addition, the linear property of INB reduces statistical restrictions of ICER. Consider an example of how to calculate INB. Katon et al[15] estimated that an enhanced treatment program targeted at depression among diabetes patients resulted in 115.4 incremental depression-free days at an incremental cost of $25. Given the patients' WTP for treatment to relieve depressive symptoms estimated to be approximately $10, they reported that the INB is $1129 (95% confidence interval, $692–$1572), calculated as (115.4 × 10 − 25). However, calculating INB involves making an assumption of monetary value placed on health benefits, which is considered a major limitation of INB by some researcher.[16]

Sensitivity Analysis

Even if the base case analysis is constructed on all of the expected values of the variables, the calculated total costs, ICER, and INB might not represent the true expected value of the measure. First, the model structure might not be able to simulate the cost and health outcomes accurately and completely. In other words, the mathematical relation between the input and output might not represent the true mechanisms in the real world. This uncertainty has been termed internal uncertainty or first-order uncertainty[17] in CEA. Second, the model outcome $f(b)$, which could be ICER or INB, is likely to be a nonlinear function of model inputs b. The expected value of $f(b)$ will not be equal to the function of the expected valued of b; that is, $E[f(b)] = f(E[b])$ does not apply in this case.

The uncertainty surrounding the variables might be traced back to different sources. First, the efficacy data obtained from one RCT might differ from another RCT conducted in different populations or with different experimental design. For example, measures of outcomes are often subjective in nature. Second, the cost estimate might only represent the average level and ignore the extreme values. Third, some values are just obtained through educated guesses or expert panel without strong empirical evidence.

Therefore, it is necessary to investigate whether any alternative data or methodology would change the base case result. The first type of uncertainty is termed *first-order uncertainty* in CEA,[17] while the uncertainty associated with variation in the values of parameters is called *second-order uncertainty*. Most of the literature thus far has reported sensitivity analysis (SA) results addressing second-order uncertainty. The following sections will focus on second-order uncertainty and discuss first-order uncertainty briefly.

Deterministic SA   Deterministic SAs include 1-way SA, multiple 1-way SA, and 2-way SA. In 1-way SA, the analysis will be repetitively conducted based on different values within the specified range for each variable, while holding all of the other variables constant at base case value. This helps identify the individual impact of the variables on the results. In contrast, multiple 1-way SA provides a comprehensive way to compare the relative impact of the variables on the results, although these are also limited to what happens when only 1 input variable changes at a time. Two-way SA is used to examine the impact on a decision of simultaneous changes in the values of 2 variables.

Probabilistic SA   The disadvantage of deterministic SAs is that they are all based on point estimates using the upper and lower bound, ignoring the varying likelihood of different values and correlation among variables. Compared to deterministic analysis, probabilistic SA (PSA) allows for the facts that all of the variables change simultaneously relative to the base case analysis and that different values for each variable will occur with varying likelihood depending on the distribution specified.

Data Collection for SA   To conduct deterministic analysis, it is important to specify the plausible range for input parameters (ie, the upper and lower bound values). However, there is no universal standard set as to how to determine the plausible range for variables. It is usually recommended to determine the range by reviewing the literature, consulting expert opinions, or using a specified confidence interval around the mean.[18] Researchers should avoid choosing ranges that are unjustifiably small for the purpose of demonstrating the robustness of estimates.

Depending on the nature of the data, uniform, normal, triangular, beta, log-normal, and gamma distributions have been assigned to different variables examined in PSA in

CEA. For example, a beta distribution might be used to fit the binomial data, such as the incidence of disease or other events. Both log-normal and gamma distributions can be used to fit cost data that can be highly skewed. However, there might be situations where assuming a statistical distribution might be too restrictive due to lack of sufficient evidence. In this case, the nonparametric bootstrapping strategy is usually recommended. However, the downside of this approach is that raw data are required.

Interpretations of SA Results   Tornado diagrams are usually used to present the results from multiple 1-way SA, providing considerable insights into the relative impact of variables on the results. In the graph, a horizontal bar is displayed for each variable, with the width of the bar representing incremental values in the outcome being evaluated corresponding to the change in the variable being analyzed. The widest bar is located on the top, with the narrowest at the bottom, indicating that the wider the bar, the larger the potential effect on the expected value of the model. As a result, a funnel-like (or Tornado like) appearance forms when all bars are arranged in the descending order of the bar width. For example, Oba[19] identified that utility weight has the largest impact on ICER of salmeterol versus no treatment, followed by mortality rate, cost of drug, and hospitalization rate. Specifically, when the quarterly mortality rate was varied from 0.97% to 1.46%, ICER ranged from $42,204 to $93,120 per quality-adjusted life-year (QALY) gained.

Cost-effectiveness acceptability curves (CEACs) are a commonly used visual tool to illustrate the impact of uncertainty on the results. The widely used CEAC in the existing literature for comparing more than 2 strategies under consideration is based on INB.[20] For example, if the PSA was based on 10,000 iterations, an INB is obtained for each of the iterations for each alternative. Each time, the option with the highest INB is identified. The probability that the option is selected as cost effective is thus equivalent to the proportion of the 10,000 iterations for which each option has the highest net benefit. Therefore, AC shows the probability that the new therapy will be cost effective as a function of the societal WTP (for a QALY) threshold. ICER helps to overcome the problems of constructing CEA confidence intervals. Apart from that, the main advantage is that it offers a natural and intuitive interpretation for decision makers: "How likely is it that the intervention will be cost effective?"

Graphically, the ICER will be displayed in the two-dimensional diagram with the horizontal axis indicating the WTP and the vertical axis indicating the probability of the examined strategy considered as cost-effective.

However, it is important to keep in mind the limitations of CEAC when communicating the results as information to be used by decision makers. Some researchers[21] have pointed out the following caveats associated with CEAC. First, because CEAC do not report which alternative has the maximum expected benefit given the WTP, it is important to note that the alternative with the maximum probability of having the maximum benefit is not necessarily the alternative with the maximum expected benefit. Second, it has been argued that CEAC provides initial insight into the evaluation of the need of further research in a sense that a probability of 65% being cost effective may suggest the need for more research, whereas 99% may suggest minimal value from more research. Despite this, it could be misleading for decision makers because CEAC are not informative as to the consequences of not selecting the "true" preferred alternative. Finally, it is difficult to synthesize results from ACs with other evidence because of a lack of a measure of the precision of the AC estimates.

Incremental cost-effectiveness (ICE) scatter plot is another way to reflect the simulation results from PSA. The scatter plot uses the cost-effectiveness plane (as shown in Figure 13-1) to plot the incremental cost and effectiveness pairs for each simulation. As a result, the ICE scatter plot demonstrates a set of points for each recalculation of the model. Thus, the incremental joint distribution in the four quadrants gives an unbiased impression of the actual value of expected costs and effects, as well as their uncertainty interval. If the simulation results tend to be concentrated below WTP line in Quadrant I as opposed above WTP line or in Quadrant IV, there are less uncertainties with the choice of the evaluated therapy as the cost-effective strategy.

Summary

Overall, CEA has been considered a powerful method in the area of health technology assessment, by which the researcher can identify, measure, and compare resources consumed for a certain level of outcomes. However, to generate meaningful information using CEA for health policy makers, it is important for analysts to follow rigorous research methodology, including data quality, model design, and results interpretation. In addition, to reduce the challenges in disseminating the results to relevant policy makers, it is critical for analysts to increase the transparency of the methodology and improve the understanding of the results by keeping the method as simple as possible without sacrificing its scientific rigor.

■ Cost-Utility Analysis

Cost-utility analysis (CUA) has been considered by some as a subset of CEA because the major difference between CUA and CEA is that the final outcomes in CUA are assessed using a special type of clinical outcome measure, usually QALYs. CUA accounts for not only life span, but also the quality of patients' life by measuring patient preferences for various health consequences, also referred to as utilities. However, the term utility might have different meanings for different people depending on their research fields.[16] It is generally considered equivalent to personal preferences; thus, it is sometimes referred to using other terms, such as *preference weight* or *preference value* in place of the word *utility*.

The measurement of QALYs covers both the benefits and possible harm of interventions to the patients and can be evaluated for a wide range of diseases and treatments. As a result, QALYs provide a means to establish the relative efficiency of various interventions. Therefore, one of the unique advantages of a CUA is that it facilitates comparison of different types of health outcomes and disease by mapping multiple outcomes of interests into one common unit: the QALY. In addition, QALY incorporates morbidity and mortality into this one common unit but eliminates the need to determine or estimate the monetary value of the health outcomes, which often involves intricate ethic issues.

Use of QALYs might not be necessary when the outcomes of interest are solely the number of years patients will live. However, use of QALYs is necessary in the situation where a therapy being evaluated might extend patients' life span but at the expense of unpleasant side effects. There are also situations when the primary outcome of interest is a patient's life quality rather than mortality. For example, in comparing alternative interventions for the treatment of arthritis,[22] the focus is usually on how well the different interventions improve the patient's regular daily physical function and overall psychological well-being. CUA has been used for other disease states such as uterine fibroids,[23] metastatic spinal tumors,[24] cervical cancer vaccination,[25] and hepatitis C.[26]

The disadvantage of this method is that it is difficult to determine an accurate utility or QALY value from a certain perspective, either the patients' perspective or the societal perspective. Although QALYs can be determined by proposed methods such as rating scale, standard gamble, and time trade-off (readers are referred to Drummond et al[18] for more details), it is not straightforward to conduct a study among patients to derive those values. This type of study involves enrolling a group of patients with moderate sample size and selecting an appropriate instrument to solicit patients' preference.

For example, to derive the QALY associated with the functional capacity for patients with rheumatoid arthritis in a CUA study,[21] patients were first asked to described their quality of life using the EuroQol (EQ)-5D and the Short Form-36 questionnaires,[27,28] from which the British and Dutch EQ-5D utilities and the Short Form-6D (SF-6D) utility[29-31] are calculated. These utilities were considered appropriate for economic evaluations from a societal perspective, but were not necessarily concordant with utilities evaluated from the patients' perspective. Thus, the investigators then obtained valuations from the patients' perspective using the time trade-off (TTO) method,[32] in which patients were asked to report how many years in optimal health they would consider equivalent to their current health for their remaining life expectancy. The TTO utility score was then calculated as the ratio of both lifetimes, suggesting the trade-off in life-years they are willing to make between current health states and optimal health. Finally, to obtain the utility curve over time used to calculate QALYs, the EQ-5D and SF-6D were assessed every 3 months, and the TTO was assessed at 0, 6, 12, and 24 months.

The amount of research effort to conduct CUA can be daunting in terms of time and personnel, which partly explains why this relatively new type of outcome measure has not been fully embraced by more US providers and decision makers (eg, payers). Therefore, although the number of CUA research articles in the literature is increasing yearly, most of the publications using this method still include the specific clinical outcome in the analysis along with QALYs. For example, Brown et al[33] reported the

ICER for each headache attack averted per month due to use of prophylactic medications along with the ICER for QALY.

Methods

The methods for CUA have many similarities to those for CEA, and all the principles discussed in the section on CEA are also applied in CUA. Generally speaking, these analyses can be considered identical on the cost side. However, a few minor differences between CUA and CEA should be kept in mind.

1. In CEA, as mentioned earlier, the ICERs are usually expressed as cost per unit of effect because the health effects are measured in natural units related to the program being evaluated. In CUA, the ICERs are usually expressed as the cost for per QALY gained.
2. Both CEA and CUA require valid effectiveness data, but CUA requires the final outcome because it is hard to establish the link between QALY and the intermediate outcomes.
3. Uncertainty associated with the measure of QALYs can often critically impact the decision of the optimal treatment strategy. Therefore, sensitivity analysis is often needed to examine whether the findings of CUA are robust to changes in QALY. For example, in a CUA study of vesicoureteral reflux, Hsieh et al[34] found that the utility penalties for invasive imaging and outpatient pyelonephritis episodes were critical in determining the highest utility treatment protocol. Similarly, a review study[35] of economic evaluations of migraine pharmacotherapy also concluded that most studies found that the choice of the optimal pharmacotherapy is sensitive to the measure of health utility gain associated with less frequency of headache.

Summary

As described, CUA requires extra effort on the part of analysts to collect data related to QALYs. One of the benefits of CUA versus CEA is that it provides a common metric of the value of the health technology and pharmaceutical. However, it may add another source of parameter uncertainty in the analysis. Therefore, it is important to evaluate the associated uncertainty in the CUA.

■ Cost-Benefit Analysis

Cost-benefit analysis (CBA) is another commonly used method in health care program evaluations. Its theoretical roots can be traced back to welfare economics.[16] Since CBA was first used in evaluating water projects such as irrigating and flood control in the 1800s and 1900s from the point of view of public health policy makers, it has become an appealing tool for setting policies related to public goods such as wildlife, air quality, public parks, and health care. The need to evaluate these types of programs arises primarily from budget constraints faced by policy makers in various areas in allocating resources to different competitive projects. In today's society, this is exactly the situation faced by health care decision makers who try to maximize health gain for the community.

As the costs of health care continue to increase, many decision makers must make choices regarding which health intervention programs such as drug therapy or medical device will be implemented. For example, pharmacists are providing clinical services or developing specialty clinical services in many areas of health care such as anticoagulation, diabetes, asthma, and human immunodeficiency virus (HIV). Although various clinical pharmacy programs might have potential in improving clinical outcomes, such as glycemic control and bone density, pressures of limited resources are forcing decision makers to consider which individual intervention has benefits that outweigh the costs or which intervention will provide the greatest benefit given a certain amount of investment. For example, CBA has been used to compare internal fixation with hemiarthroplasty in the treatment for displaced femoral neck fractures in elderly patients,[36] in studies evaluating whether it is worth the cost for pregnant women to undergo thrombophilia screening,[37] and in studies evaluating the use of biopsy along with brachytherapy in the treatment of localized prostate cancer.[38]

One of the advantages of CBA studies is that the results can be represented as benefit-to-cost ratio, which helps decision makers determine which program's costs exceed the benefits and to what degree. If the goal of the decision maker is to maximize the monetary return from the investment, the program with the highest benefit-to-cost ratio would be chosen. In addition, it is impossible to compare the value of the various interventions if only the CER from CEA or CUA were available. CBA also expands the scope of the programs being evaluated by allowing comparison between interventions in health care and those in different sectors of the economy. In contrast, CEA and CUA are restricted to the comparison of health care interventions because they are analyzed with outcomes restricted to health benefits.

However, the unique requirements of placing a monetary value on the outcomes of CBA also pose a challenge in real-world analysis. For example, comparing programs that can reduce mortality rates for children and for adults gives rise to controversies regarding how much a human life at different stages is worth in monetary terms. There is no standard agreement about how to measure the benefits and what benefits should be included. For instance, as argued by Labelle and Hurley,[39] it might be necessary to take into account the externalities of the effects of a health intervention, which can be positive or negative. Consider HIV or the common flu as an example. The benefit gained by one individual can have multiplying benefits to other individuals. In theory, it is possible to capture such effects, but in practice, this has not yet been done. There are 3 general approaches to the monetary valuation of health outcomes: (1) human capital, (2) revealed preferences, and (3) stated preferences of WTP. Readers are referred to Drummond et al[18] for more details.

Method

CEA and CUA can be considered as subtypes of CBA, where the outcomes or benefits of a health intervention or pharmaceutical are measured as physical units and health utility, respectively, as opposed to monetary value adopted by CBA. Therefore, the methods for CBA share considerable similarity with those for CEA and CUA. For example, like CEA or CUA, CBA also involves identifying the types of costs associated with a program once the program or intervention being evaluated has been determined. For example, in a CBA study that examined whether the benefit of launching a bloodstream infection control program in general hospitals in Canada justifies the cost,[40] the costs identified in the study primarily included investment costs of establishing and maintaining an infection control program in a hospital including personnel resources, such as a hospital epidemiologist, an infection control practitioner, and support personnel, and nonpersonnel resources, such as office support, computing support, audiovisual support, microbiology laboratory support, pathology services, and reference laboratory testing.

It is also important to specify the perspective of the CBA because one factor considered to be a benefit from one perspective may be a cost from another perspective. For example, providing transportation to hospitals for patients will increase patients' access to health care services but will impose a financial burden to the provider or payer. Similarly, health program benefits cannot be reaped until the program has been in place for a sustained period of time (years or decades); therefore, it is necessary to compare the discounted future streams of incremental monetary return with incremental costs. Results in CBA will be reported either using benefit-to-cost ratio or net benefits. Benefit-to-cost ratio is obtained by dividing the net present monetary value of the health benefits (denoted by B) by the net present value of the total investment (denoted by C) in the health program calculated using a discount rate. Net benefits are obtained by subtracting C from B. The goal of analysis is to identify whether an intervention's benefits exceed its costs; a positive net social benefit or a benefit-to-cost ratio greater than unity indicates that an intervention is worthwhile.

Summary

In terms of reporting results, because a large benefit-to-cost ratio will be a result of lower cost or an enormous amount of benefit, this formulation is often considered as problematic. Caution should be exercised in interpretation of the results of CBA, and special attention should be paid to the relative magnitude of benefits and costs. The precise decision rule for CBA will depend on the context of the evaluation.[18] Finally, in CBA, both costs and benefits are measured in dollar values. This can sometimes cause confusion because benefits are also costs saved.

■ References

1. Pandharipande PV, Gervais DA, Mueller PR, et al. Radiofrequency ablation versus nephron-sparing surgery for small unilateral renal cell carcinoma: cost-effectiveness analysis. *Radiology.* 2008;248:169–178.

2. Perfetto EM, Weiss KA, Mullins CD, et al. An economic evaluation of triptan products for migraine. *Value Health.* 2005;8:647–655.

3. Johansson P, Ostenson C, Hilding A, et al. A cost-effectiveness analysis of a community-based diabetes prevention program in Sweden. *Int J Technol Assess Health Care.* 2009;25:350–358.

4. Brown JS, Papadopoulos G, Neumann PJ, et al. Cost-effectiveness of migraine prevention: the case of topiramate in the UK. *Cephalalgia.* 2006;26:1473–1482.

5. Spencer M, Briggs A, Grossman R, et al. Development of an economic model to assess the cost effectiveness of treatment interventions for chronic obstructive pulmonary disease. *Pharmacoeconomics.* 2005;23:619–637.

6. Liew D, Lim S, Bertram M, et al. A model for undertaking effectiveness and cost-effectiveness analyses of primary preventive strategies in cardiovascular disease. *Eur J Cardiovasc Prev Rehabil.* 2006;13:515–522.

7. Kelman L, Von Seggern RL. Using patient-centered endpoints to determine the cost-effectiveness of triptans for acute migraine therapy. *Am J Ther.* 2006;13:411–417.

8. Gold MR, Russell LB, Weinstein MC, eds. *Time Preference in Cost-Effectiveness in Health and Medicine.* New York, NY: Oxford University Press; 1996:214–235.

9. Koopmanschap MA, Rutten F, van Ineveld B, et al. The friction cost method for measuring indirect costs of disease. *J Health Econ.* 1995;14:171–189.

10. Soto J. Health economic evaluations using decision analytic modeling. Principles and practices—utilization of a checklist to their development and appraisal. *Int J Technol Assess Health Care.* 2002;18:94–111.

11. Bodger K, Kikuchi T, Hughes D. Cost-effectiveness of biological therapy for Crohn's disease: Markov cohort analyses incorporating United Kingdom patient-level cost data. *Aliment Pharmacol Ther.* 2009;30:265–274.

12. Sher DJ, Wittenberg E, Taghian A, et al. Partial breast irradiation versus whole breast radiotherapy for early-stage breast cancer: a decision analysis. *Int J Radiat Oncol Biol Phys.* 2008;70:469–476.

13. Buti M, Brosa M, Casado M, et al. Modeling the cost-effectiveness of different oral antiviral therapies in patients with chronic hepatitis B. *J Hepatol.* 2009;51:640–646.

14. Stinnett AA, Mullahy J. Net health benefits: a new framework for the analysis of uncertainty in cost-effectiveness analysis. *Med Decis Making.* 1998;18(Suppl 2):S68–S80.

15. Katon W, Unützer J, Fan MY, et al. Cost-effectiveness and net benefit of enhanced treatment of depression for older adults with diabetes and depression. *Diabetes Care.* 2006;29:265–270.

16. Rascati KL. *Essentials of Pharmacoeconomics.* Philadelphia, PA: Lippincott Williams & Wilkins; 2008.

17. Briggs A, Sculpher M. *Decision Modelling for Health Economic Evaluation.* Oxford, UK: Oxford University Press; 2006.

18. Drummond MF, Sculpher M, Torrance GW, et al. *Methods for the Economic Evaluation of Health Care Programmes.* Oxford, UK: Oxford Medical Publications; 1997.

19. Oba Y. Cost-effectiveness of salmeterol, fluticasone, and combination therapy for COPD. *Am J Manag Care.* 2009;15:226–232.

20. Barton GR, Briggs AH, Fenwick EA. Optimal cost-effectiveness decisions: the role of the cost-effectiveness acceptability curve (CEAC), the cost-effectiveness acceptability frontier (CEAF), and the expected value of perfection information (EVPI). *Value Health*. 2008;11:886–897.

21. Groot Koerkamp B, Hunink M, Stijnen T, et al. Limitations of acceptability curves for presenting uncertainty in cost-effectiveness analysis. *Med Decis Making*. 2007;27:101–111.

22. van den Hout WB, Goekoop-Ruiterman YP, Allaart CF, et al. Cost-utility analysis of treatment strategies in patients with recent-onset rheumatoid arthritis. *Arthritis Rheum*. 2009;61:291–299.

23. You JH, Sahota DS, Yuen PM. Uterine artery embolization, hysterectomy, or myomectomy for symptomatic uterine fibroids: a cost-utility analysis. *Fertil Steril*. 2009;91:580–588.

24. Papatheofanis FJ, Williams E, Chang SD. Cost-utility analysis of the cyberknife system for metastatic spinal tumors. *Neurosurgery*. 2009;64(Suppl 2):A73–A83.

25. Anonychuk AM, Bauch C, Merid M, et al. A cost-utility analysis of cervical cancer vaccination in preadolescent Canadian females. *BMC Public Health*. 2009;9:401.

26. Sutton AJ, Edmunds W, Sweeting M, et al. The cost-effectiveness of screening and treatment for hepatitis C in prisons in England and Wales: a cost-utility analysis. *J Viral Hepat*. 2008;15:797–808.

27. The EuroQol Group. EuroQol—a new facility for the measurement of health-related quality of life. *Health Policy*. 1990;16:199–208.

28. Hays RD, Sherbourne CD, Mazel RM. The RAND 36-Item Health Survey 1.0. *Health Econ*. 1993;2:217–227.

29. Dolan P. Modeling valuations for EuroQol health states. *Med Care*. 1997;35:1095–1108.

30. Lamers LM, Stalmeier PF, McDonnell J, et al. [Measuring the quality of life in economic evaluations: the Dutch EQ-5D tariff.] *Ned Tijdschr Geneeskd*. 2005;149:1574–1578.

31. Brazier J, Czoski-Murray C, Roberts J, et al. Estimation of a preference-based index from a condition-specific measure: the King's Health Questionnaire. *Med Decis Making*. 2008;28:113–126.

32. Tijhuis GJ, Jansen SJ, Stiggelbout AM, et al. Value of the time trade off method for measuring utilities in patients with rheumatoid arthritis. *Ann Rheum Dis*. 2000;59:892–897.

33. Brown JS, Papadopoulos G, Neumann PJ, et al. Cost-effectiveness of topiramate in migraine prevention: results from a pharmacoeconomic model of topiramate treatment. *Headache*. 2005;45:1012–1022.

34. Hsieh MH, Swana HS, Baskin LS, et al. Cost-utility analysis of treatment algorithms for moderate grade vesicoureteral reflux using Markov models. *J Urol*. 2007;177:703–709.

35. Yu J, Goodman MJ, Oderda GM. Economic evaluation of pharmacotherapy of migraine pain: a review of the literature. *J Pain Palliat Care Pharmacother*. 2009;23:396–408.

36. Alolabi B, Bajammal S, Shirali J, et al. Treatment of displaced femoral neck fractures in the elderly: a cost-benefit analysis. *J Orthop Trauma*. 2009;23:442–446.

37. Salvagno GL, Lippi G, Franchini M, et al. The cost-benefit ratio of screening pregnant women for thrombophilia. *Blood Transfus*. 2007;5:189–203.

38. Cambio AJ, Ellison LM, Chamie K, et al. Cost-benefit and outcome analysis: effect of prostate biopsy undergrading. *Urology*. 2007;69:1152–1156.

39. Labelle RJ, Hurley JE. Implications of basing health-care resource allocations on cost-utility analysis in the presence of externalities. *J Health Econ*. 1992;11:259–277.

40. Hong Z, Wu J, Tisdell C, et al. Cost-benefit analysis of preventing nosocomial bloodstream infections among hemodialysis patients in Canada in 2004. *Value Health*. 2010;13:42–45.

Comparative Effectiveness

Patrick D. Meek, PharmD, MSPH
Amy C. Renaud-Mutart, PharmD, MSPharm
Leon E. Cosler, RPh, PhD

Learning Objectives

- Define comparative effectiveness research.

- Describe the various forms of comparative effectiveness research.

- Compare and contrast comparative effectiveness analyses with other techniques such as cost-benefit or cost-effectiveness analyses.

- Describe situations in which comparative effectiveness analyses, including evaluations of cost, would be the optimal analytical technique.

- Discuss how comparative effectiveness analyses may help control US health care costs.

- Understand the arguments for and against establishing a national center for comparative effectiveness in the United States.

- Discuss how comparative effectiveness analyses could be integrated into pharmaceutical research and clinical pharmacy practice.

■ Introduction

In 2009, the US Department of Health and Human Services held the first of three public listening sessions in Washington, DC, to discuss the use of comparative effectiveness research (CER) in health care. This meeting followed an announcement that a committee called the Federal Coordinating Council for Comparative Effectiveness Research had been established to coordinate research and guide investments in comparative effectiveness research as directed by the Recovery Act. Stimulated by the 2009 American Recovery and Reinvestment Act (www.hhs.gov/recovery/programs/cer/), a total of $1.1 billion has been allocated over a 2-year period. The Council achieved several developmental goals and was sunsetted (with a planned termination) in March 2010. Upon passage of the Patient Protection and Affordable Care Act of 2010, the Patient Centered Outcomes Research

Institute (PCORI), a national center for Comparative Effectiveness Research was established to replace the Council.

CER is defined by the Institute of Medicine (IOM) as "the generation and synthesis of evidence that compares the benefits and harms of alternative methods to prevent, diagnose, treat and monitor a clinical condition, or to improve the delivery of care."[1] Stated differently, CER aims to judge relevant treatment options (head-to-head) for a specified condition or disease state and to develop evidence that assists consumers, clinicians, purchasers, and policy makers to make informed decisions that will improve health care at both the individual and population levels (ie, "decision-based evidence making"). To fully understand the potential impact of CER, it is helpful to understand what this research entails and how it could potentially be used to reshape the structure of our health care system.

■ Background on CER

The basic premise behind CER is to provide health care decision makers with appropriate, relevant data on the outcomes of commonly prescribed therapies to guide the selection of the most effective treatments. For example, a CER study might evaluate the results of surgery versus medication for a given condition or how patients with high cholesterol respond to similar drugs such as Lipitor, Zocor, and Crestor. The origins of CER date back to the late 1970s, so it is not a new concept. Regrettably, much of the early media coverage surrounding this subject neglected to mention how CER positively impacts health care practice. For example, the guidelines for treating newly diagnosed cases of hypertension were revised largely due to the findings of CER-based studies. The research showed that the most effective way to begin treatment of patients with hypertension is with a generic diuretic and a β-blocker—at a cost of only pennies per day. This finding has had a major influence on how patients with hypertension are treated, resulting in improved care at a lower cost.

In the absence of CER data, practitioners are often forced to rely on the results of clinical trials to help make decisions on the best ways to treat patients, but this information has severe limitations. This is because the drug approval process in the United States essentially requires that a given treatment work better than nothing (ie, a placebo) and that it is generally found to be safe and effective in the well-controlled environment of clinical trials. It does not require proof that a treatment works better than, or even as good as, well-accepted standards.

The reality is that health care practitioners treat patients with a variety of complex conditions, as opposed to the carefully screened individuals who participate in trials. For that reason, CER is widely recognized as filling a critical gap in the collective knowledge base by providing data on the success or failure of treatment options administered in a more generalizeable clinical practice. It is when the discussion shifts to how CER data should be used to make payment decisions that opinions begin to quickly diverge among practitioners, patients, payers, and manufacturers of medical therapies including pharmaceutical companies.

This chapter aims to present the basic philosophy behind CER and to introduce the reader to principles and terminology that will be encountered in the CER literature. We include a review of common research designs and some of the basic principles of economic analysis of health care interventions and discuss how these techniques fit in with the field of CER. We also provide a global perspective of CER by reviewing programs from other countries that aim to guide health care policy through evidence development. Lastly, we conclude the chapter with a summary of CER and implications for the practice of clinical pharmacy.

■ Forms of CER

CER can take many forms and draw from many types of research designed to compare alternative treatment options, including prospective observational or experimental studies, systematic reviews and meta-analyses, retrospective studies with existing data, and simulation modeling (with or without cost data). Several examples of highly cited prospective comparative effectiveness studies exist in the literature (TABLE 14-1). These trials have a number of characteristics in common: (1) inclusion of the most common and clinically reasonable treatment alternatives for each condition; (2) comparison of outcomes of interest to clinicians; (3) adequate duration of follow-up; and (4) enrollment of populations that are likely to be encountered in actual clinical practice.

Pragmatic trials are a type of clinical trial that aims to test whether a treatment is effective in real-life situations. When practical aspects of treatment, such as compliance, are relevant to treatment decisions, pragmatic clinical trials allow for treatments to run a natural course, and the flexibility of the trial design maintains validity of comparison through the use of specialized pragmatic trial techniques. In contrast to traditional clinical trials, the design of a pragmatic trial reflects variations between patients that occur in actual clinical practice, such as variation in treatment adherence, and aims to inform choices between treatments, accounting for this variation.

Other prospective trials that are used in the field of CER and warrant description include *cluster randomized trials* and *delayed-start design trials*. Unlike randomized trials, which randomly allocate treatment at the level of the individual patient, cluster randomized trials allocate treatment of study participants at the site level. This is favorable when comparing treatment interventions that are part of a treatment program and are not restricted to a single drug or therapy. Delayed-start design trials are studies that randomize patients to immediate versus delayed treatment. This method has been implemented in diseases, such as Parkinson disease and other movement disorders, in which treatment benefit is measured in terms of progression times, rather than cure or resolution of disease.

Reviews of existing research are also an important way to summarize available evidence about the benefits and harms of alternative treatment choices. Evidence from available clinical trials forms the basis for treatment decisions and, when summarized systematically, can yield valuable insight into the benefits of available alternatives and bring to light gaps in the current knowledge about the most effective treatment

Table 14-1	Examples of Published Comparative Effectiveness Studies

Antihypertensive and Lipid-Lowering Treatment to Prevent Heart Attack Trial (ALLHAT)[2-4]

Rationale/aims	(1) To determine whether newer types of antihypertensive agents are as good as or better than diuretics in reducing coronary heart disease incidence and progression; (2) to determine whether lowering low-density lipoprotein cholesterol in moderately hypercholesterolemic older individuals will reduce the incidence of cardiovascular disease and total mortality. Both aims were evaluated over a 6-year follow-up period.
Study design	Randomized double-blind trial designed to evaluate whether outcomes differ between persons randomized to diuretic treatment and each of 3 alternative treatments: a calcium channel blocker, an angiotensin-converting enzyme inhibitor, and an α-adrenergic blocker; ALLHAT also contained an open-label, randomized trial of lipid-lowering therapy in the subset of patients with high cholesterol to evaluate HMG-CoA treatment compared with "usual care."
Study population	40,000 high-risk hypertensive patients with 1 or more additional risk factor for heart attack and who were at least 55 years of age
Significance of results	Confirmed the significance of thiazide diuretics for patients older than age 55 years
Conclusions	Cheap diuretics are just as effective as more expensive agents for first-line treatment of hypertension.

Sudden Cardiac Death Heart Failure Trial (SCD-HeFT)[5]

Rationale/aims	To determine whether amiodarone and/or implantable cardioverter-defibrillator (ICD) therapy for primary prevention of sudden cardiac death improves overall survival compared with placebo during a minimum of 2.5 years of follow-up.
Study design	Randomized, placebo-controlled trial
Study population	Patients with mild-to-moderate clinical symptoms of congestive heart failure (New York Heart Association Class II or III) and significantly decreased left ventricular ejection fraction
Significance of results	The SCD-HeFT results show that ICDs save the lives of people with moderate heart failure and poor heart pumping function, due to their risk of sudden cardiac arrest (SCA).
	Because SCA is responsible for 60% of deaths among Americans with heart failure, the findings from the trial also reinforce the importance of receiving ICD therapy as a preventative measure before experiencing an episode of SCA.
	Amiodarone, an oral medication previously believed to be the "gold standard" antiarrhythmic drug, was shown to be ineffective in preventing sudden cardiac death. This reinforces the fact that defibrillation is the only treatment that can stop a life-threatening heart rhythm once it occurs.
	SCD-HeFT is the largest and longest follow-up ICD trial ever conducted. Most previous heart failure ICD trials studied therapy among the most

(continues)

Table 14-1	Examples of Published Comparative Effectiveness Studies (Continued)
	severe heart failure patients and had shorter follow-up periods. SCD-HeFT was designed to look at a broader class of heart failure patients and follow them longer with a control group more than twice the size of any previous heart failure trial.
	SCD-HeFT is the latest in a series of major medical studies demonstrating the life-saving benefits of ICDs. The results reinforce evidence from earlier trials (eg, MADIT, MUSTT, and MADIT II) that showed that ICDs significantly cut the risk of death (31%–55%) in certain groups of heart attack survivors.
Conclusions	In patients with heart failure, defibrillators save lives, whereas the medication amiodarone does not.

Diabetes Prevention Program (DPP) Trial[6,7]

Rationale/aims	To determine whether prevention (through lifestyle modification) rather than early detection and treatment of diabetes might be more effective in preventing diabetes and microvascular and macrovascular complications
Study design	Randomized, placebo-controlled trial with 3–5 years of follow-up to evaluate differences in diabetes incidence between individuals randomized to metformin, lifestyle modification, or placebo
Study population	High-risk, nondiabetic individuals over age 25 years with elevated fasting plasma glucose concentrations and impaired glucose tolerance
Significance of results	The DPP found that participants who lost a modest amount of weight through dietary changes and increased physical activity sharply reduced their chances of developing diabetes. Taking metformin also reduced risk, although less dramatically.
Conclusions	Lifestyle changes are superior to medication in preventing or slowing the onset of diabetes.

Clinical Antipsychotic Trials of Intervention Effectiveness (CATIE)[8]

Rationale/aims	Pragmatic clinical trial
Study design	Randomized, multicenter trial of ziprasidone, risperidone, quetiapine, olanzapine, and perphenazine with follow-up for 18 months, followed by trial pathways in which medications can be discontinued before participants are randomized to further treatment arms. In the third phase, participants could choose from 1 of 9 treatment pathways. Time to discontinuation of treatment was the primary outcome.
Study population	Adults with chronic schizophrenia
Significance of results	The trial was designed to examine fundamental issues about second-generation antipsychotic medications (olanzapine, risperidone, quetiapine, and ziprasidone), including their relative effectiveness and their effectiveness compared to a first-generation antipsychotic, perphenazine.
Conclusions	The older antipsychotic medication perphenazine is less expensive and no less effective than newer medications.

HMG-CoA, 3-hydroxy-3-methyl-glutaryl–conenzyme A.

alternatives. Systematic reviews and meta-analyses provide valuable information pertaining to the likelihood of achieving desired outcomes and may be useful for simulation studies when data from empirically designed trials are not available.

Simulation or modeling studies are another form of research that may be used in CER. These techniques use statistical methods for deriving estimates of the probabilities of treatment outcomes given the evidence about treatment effectiveness, safety, and costs. Simulation studies may use information from systematic reviews or from other existing data derived from health care databases, such as claims data or electronic medical record data.

■ CER and Analytic Techniques Involving Costs

Although the current IOM definition of comparative effectiveness does not specifically mention the comparison of costs of therapy, it is anticipated that a comparison of costs will be one of the major metrics used by constituents such as health care purchasers (as well as others) conducting CER. Thus, the traditional health technology assessment techniques involving the assessment of costs (eg, cost-benefit analysis, cost-effectiveness analysis) can be expected to play a major role in CER. Therefore, it is important to understand the roles of these designs in the larger milieu of CER.

CER typically will not include descriptive cost studies, such as cost-of-illness or cost-of-episode analyses because these designs typically do not use comparators of health care interventions. Rather, the key economic designs expected to play a role in CER include cost-benefit analysis, cost-effectiveness analysis, and cost-utility analysis. It should be noted that these evaluation designs can be used both in the randomized clinical trial setting and in nonrandomized, observational designs. It is important to keep in mind that CER studies focus exclusively on comparisons conducted in real-world, non-randomized environments.

Cost-benefit analysis (CBA) designs typically require that resources and benefits are both valued in the same metric, typically dollars or other local currency. For example, if the therapeutic intervention is shown to save or extend years of life, these years must be valued in dollar terms. Because of this requirement, which can be onerous and sometimes controversial, CBA has had relatively limited use in economic assessments of health care interventions. CBA can be used to evaluate single programs (comparing net costs to net benefits) or to compare multiple programs for the greatest net benefit. Because of the requirement of resources and outcomes expressed in one financial metric, the greatest usefulness for CBA is its ability to be used to compare very disparate interventions or programs, where the health outcomes may be vastly different, but a decision maker is faced with making an allocation decision with fixed budgetary constraints. To date, the most common applications for health care–related CBA studies have been in the evaluation of vaccines, immunization programs, and antibiotic therapies.[9,10]

Cost-effectiveness analysis (CEA) is a popular and powerful technique for assessing relative costs and benefits of health care interventions. This design differs from CBA in that benefits or health outcomes are not assessed in monetary terms, but compared in their natural units (eg, years of life saved, inpatient length of stay, symptom-free days). CEA thus avoids the difficulty of placing a monetary value on human life or survival times and is easier for many health practitioners to use and interpret. The major limitation of using CEA as an assessment tool is that it can only be used to compare outcomes that are measured with the same outcome (unit of analysis). For example, therapies to reduce hypertension could not be directly compared with therapies intended to control blood glucose.

Limitations notwithstanding, the presentation and interpretation of the results of CEA will likely be very common within the field of comparative effectiveness research. Unlike CBA, which offers a single "net benefit" metric, CEA provides decision makers with a ratio of the incremental costs of 2 (or more) options per outcome measure. An option is considered cost effective when it is less costly and at least as equally effective as the comparator, or when any cost differences are offset by sufficient additional positive outcomes. Typically, strategies can be portrayed in a matrix where the choice of strategies is obvious or, more commonly, when a decision maker is required to make some trade-off decisions for additional resources necessary to adopt a more effective treatment alternative (FIGURE 14-1). It is anticipated that CER will be conducted in a way that similarly quantifies outcomes where the comparison of 2 treatment alternatives will not be obvious, but rather will be portrayed in such a way that decision makers will be able to make relevant informed decisions in the common situation that additional resources will frequently be necessary for additional gains in health outcomes.

COST EFFECTIVENESS	Lower cost	Equal cost	Higher cost
Lower effectiveness	A [conduct ICER]	B	C [dominated]
Equal effectiveness	D	E [arbitrary]	F
Higher effectiveness	G [dominant]	H	I [conduct ICER]

FIGURE 14-1 Cost-effectiveness decision grid. ICER, incremental cost-effectiveness ratio.

Source: Adapted from L Rascati, *Essentials of Pharmacoeconomics.* Lippincott: Williams & Wilkins; 2009.

Closely related to CEA designs are cost-utility analyses (CUAs). These designs evaluate the costs of different health interventions (FIGURE 14-2), but in terms of a very special denominator—a quality-adjusted clinical outcome (eg, quality-adjusted life-years [QALYs]). CUA requires that patient preferences (ie, utilities) be used to adjust the clinical outcomes being measured. The advantages of CUA are that very dissimilar health interventions can often be compared if their outcomes can be expressed in the same units (eg, QALYs). Obviously, a major hurdle in employing this technique is the ability to determine patient preferences for different states of health and well-being. However, because of the attractiveness of incorporating patient preferences, health utilities are becoming more commonplace, especially for the most common diseases. CUA holds much promise for a role in CER because of its ability to incorporate patient preferences and particularly because this design can be used to evaluate health strategies that do not affect patient survival or length of illness, but rather affect the quality of patients' lives during or after treatment. Figure 14-2 provides an illustration of the manner in which outcomes research designs may vary, based on two key characteristics (allocation method, and type of outcomes). The method of allocation is shown on the x-axis with randomized designs to the left, and non-randomized designs to the right. The type of outcome is presented on the y-axis with economic outcomes on the top, and non-economic outcomes on the bottom. This figure illustrates the relationships that exist between study designs used to evaluate comparative effectiveness.

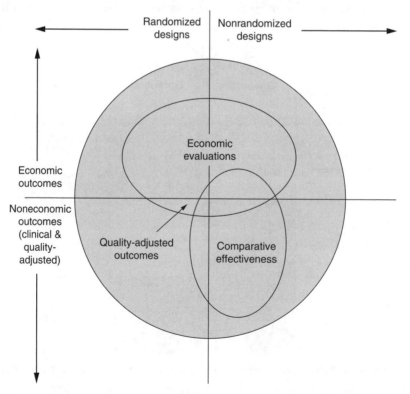

FIGURE 14-2 Contrasting randomized and nonrandomized outcomes research designs.

Situations in Which Comparative Effectiveness Analysis with an Economic Analysis Would be the Best Choice

Economics tells us that the optimal way to spend a limited amount of health care dollars is to organize care around the most cost-effective therapies. However, the best method to conduct a comparative effectiveness analysis will be driven by a number of factors, primarily the perspective of the study and whether costs are a desired outcome to be assessed. For example, oncologists who are seeking the most effective chemotherapy regimen for metastatic colorectal cancer may evaluate different therapeutic options (with or without surgical options) in terms of remission rates and patient survival rates. A comparative effectiveness analysis, in this case, may not use costs as a measured outcome. However, health insurance purchasers, conducting the same analysis, would likely be very interested in comparing costs as an important outcome and may opt for one of the economic evaluation techniques such as CEA or CUA.

■ Impact of CER in the United States

In 2007, US health care spending totaled approximately $7421 per capita, exceeding $2.2 trillion and accounting for 16.2% of gross domestic product (GDP). Health care expenditures are expected to increase at an average rate of 6.2% over the next several years and are projected to total $4.4 trillion, or 20.3% of GDP, by 2018. For comparison, GDP is expected to increase by an average of only 4.1% annually between 2008 and 2018. Obviously, this rate of growth is unsustainable over the long term.[11,12] The rapid growth in health care expenditures over the past several decades has been fueled by several factors. Advances in health technologies such as pharmaceuticals and diagnostic equipment are generally considered to be the primary drivers of cost increases. Other contributing factors include an aging population, the increasing prevalence of health insurance, and growth in average personal incomes, all of which generate heightened demand for health care goods and services. Although the United States spends more than any other nation on health care, the outcomes realized are not significantly better than those of countries with lower expenditures.[13]

Use of CER Studies in International Single-Payer and Social Insurance Health Care Models

Comparative effectiveness studies play a significant role in the health care spending budgetary decisions of nations that use single-payer or social insurance coverage models. In the United Kingdom, the National Institute for Health and Clinical Excellence (NICE) is the tax-funded organization of the single-payer National Health System (NHS) that evaluates the clinical and cost effectiveness of a wide range of medical interventions. The NICE model of CER synthesizes systematic literature reviews of clinical effectiveness trials with cost-effectiveness models to establish clinical guidelines and make coverage recommendations for all health technologies, including pharmaceuticals, medical devices, and procedures. Any intervention approved by NICE must be covered under the NHS.[14,15]

Because the NHS operates within a set budget, determining the clinical and economic effectiveness of interventions through CER is essential to its function. However, countries in which national health systems operate with open (on-demand) budgets also find CER to be a useful tool for controlling costs. For example, in Germany, the Institute for Quality and Efficiency in Health Care (IQWiG), an independent scientific institution funded by levies on health care services, investigates the economic and clinical effectiveness of a broad range of diagnostic and therapeutic interventions. Its findings are instrumental in determining what services will be covered by statutory health insurance. In contrast, the focus of the Australian CER entity is much more narrow than that of either NICE or IQWiG. The Pharmaceutical Benefits Advisory Committee, a committee of the Department of Health and Ageing, contracts with academic institutions to perform economic and clinical evaluations of drugs for inclusion on the Pharmaceutical Benefits Scheme formulary.[14,16]

Existing Capacity for CER in the United States

Several entities in both the private and public sectors in the United States already engage in some form of CER. Health insurance companies and hospitals routinely assess the economic and clinical benefits of pharmaceuticals for formulary inclusion. In 1985, the Blue Cross Blue Shield Association established the Technology Evaluation Center (TEC) to review interventions on behalf of clients for appropriateness and clinical effectiveness. The TEC includes among its clients the Centers for Medicare and Medicaid Services. In the public sector, several federal agencies engage in some form of CER or promotion.

Most notably, the Agency for Healthcare Research and Quality (AHRQ) engages in limited CER as authorized by the Medicare Prescription Drug, Improvement, and Modernization Act of 2003. The National Institutes of Health (NIH) also engages in limited CER. However, neither agency can truly be considered a center for CER, because comparative effectiveness–related activities account for only about 20% of the AHRQ budget and a small fraction of NIH expenditures.[16,17]

Proposal to Establish a Quasi-Governmental National Comparative Effectiveness Center in the United States

In 2006, Gail Wilensky, a former administrator of the Health Care Financing Administration, published a seminal paper in the journal *Health Affairs* proposing the establishment of a quasi-governmental national center for CER in the United States.[16] Such a center would compare interventions and technologies solely for the purpose of obtaining information and would make no coverage or other budgetary recommendations to any entity, public or private. The proposed center would not only serve as a clearinghouse for gathering, organizing, and disseminating existing data, but also be instrumental in the funding of prospective trials in areas for which comparative effectiveness information is determined to be lacking. Because the CER activities currently conducted by agencies such as AHRQ and NICE are generally restricted to meta-analyses of existing information, the contributions of such a center as proposed would be of enormous significance to the global community.[16]

The PCORI is an independent, non-profit organization established by the Patient Protection and Affordable Care Act of 2010 to help patients, clinicians, purchasers and policy makers make better informed health decisions. The anticipated annual PCORI budget (derived in part from a 1% tax on health care premiums) is expected to reach $500 million by 2015 and will be used to support the PCORI mission. The over arching goals of the PCORI are twofold: 1) to promote, conduct, and commission research that is responsive to the values and interests of patients and 2) to provide patients and their caregivers with high quality information for the health care choices they face.

The PCORI is governed by a 21-member Board of Governors; nineteen members appointed by the U.S. Government Accountability Office, and the directors, or their designees from the Agency for Healthcare Research and Quality (1 member) and the National Institutes of Health (1 member). The Board includes individuals representing patients and health care consumers; clinicians; private payers; manufacturers and developers of drugs, devices, and diagnostics; independent health service researchers; and leaders in federal and state health programs and agencies. The PCORI will not recommend clinical guidelines for payment, coverage or treatment rather it will consider the needs of populations served by federal programs and provide input on priorities for research funding. Findings will serve as guidance, rather than mandates, for decision makers in making health care decisions.[17,18]

Of course, there is opposition to the widespread adoption of CER for decision making and the establishment of a national center. Unlike clinical effectiveness trials, which compare similar interventions, prospective comparative effectiveness trials evaluate all available interventions for a condition. The pharmaceutical industry thus opposes the creation of a national center for CER on the basis that drug therapies have long been proven to be cost effective compared to other, more costly interventions such as surgery. There is also political and public opposition to the proposal, stemming from the perception of CER as an unacceptable step toward rationing of health care. Because the current rate of growth in US health care spending is unsustainable, however, action must be taken to control expenditures. Despite the claims of the opposition, establishing a center for CER appears to be a viable first step toward reining in costs.[18]

■ CER and Clinical Pharmacy Practice

In clinical practice, pharmacists are closely involved in treatment selection for individual patients; as such, their familiarity with evidence-based practices should include a familiarity with the area of CER. This should include skills in literature review of traditional designs and knowledge of designs relevant to the area of comparative effectiveness, including pharmacoeconomics, technology assessments, and outcomes research. Through their participation on patient care teams and on formulary committees, pharmacists serve a vital role in the clinical decision–making and drug policy–making process in which comparative effectiveness will have an impact in defining the merits of a drug in relation to other treatment alternatives.

Pharmacists may also be closely involved in the design of comparative effectiveness trials and other trials that aim to define the optimal use of drug therapy for specific patient populations in actual clinical practice. The limitations of a given trial need to be understood by those making treatment decisions. CER will not be a perfect solution in all situations, but this new area of research holds substantial promise toward closing the knowledge gap for the selection of the most effective, highest value treatment alternative.

■ References

1. Sox HC, Greenfield S. Comparative effectiveness research: a report from the Institute of Medicine. *Ann Intern Med*. 2009;151:203–205.

2. Davis BR, Cutler JA, Gordon DJ, et al. Rationale and design for the Antihypertensive and Lipid Lowering Treatment to Prevent Heart Attack Trial (ALLHAT). ALLHAT Research Group. *Am J Hypertens*. 1996;9:342–360.

3. Davis BR, Cutler JA, Furberg CD, et al. Relationship of antihypertensive treatment regimens and change in blood pressure to risk for heart failure in hypertensive patients randomly assigned to doxazosin or chlorthalidone: further analyses from the Antihypertensive and Lipid-Lowering Treatment to Prevent Heart Attack Trial. *Ann Intern Med*. 2002;137:313–320.

4. Major cardiovascular events in hypertensive patients randomized to doxazosin vs chlorthalidone: the Antihypertensive and Lipid-Lowering Treatment to Prevent Heart Attack Trial (ALLHAT). ALLHAT Collaborative Research Group. *JAMA*. 2000;283:1967–1975.

5. Bardy GH, Lee KL, Mark DB, et al. Amiodarone or an implantable cardioverter-defibrillator for congestive heart failure. *N Engl J Med*. 2005;352:225–237.

6. Knowler WC, Barrett-Connor E, Fowler SE, et al. Reduction in the incidence of type 2 diabetes with lifestyle intervention or metformin. *N Engl J Med*. 2002;346:393–403.

7. The Diabetes Prevention Program. Design and methods for a clinical trial in the prevention of type 2 diabetes. *Diabetes Care*. 1999;22:623–634.

8. Lieberman JA, Stroup TS, McEvoy JP, et al. Effectiveness of antipsychotic drugs in patients with chronic schizophrenia. *N Engl J Med*. 2005;353:1209–1223.

9. Koplan JP, Preblud SR. A benefit-cost analysis of mumps vaccine. *Am J Dis Child*. 1982;136:362–364.

10. Shapiro M, Schoenbaum SC, Tager IB, Munoz A, Polk BF. Benefit-cost analysis of antimicrobial prophylaxis in abdominal and vaginal hysterectomy. *JAMA*. 1983;249:1290–1294.

11. Hartman M, Martin A, McDonnell P, Catlin A. National health spending in 2007: slower drug spending contributes to lowest rate of overall growth since 1998. *Health Aff (Millwood)*. 2009;28:246–261.

12. Sisko A, Truffer C, Smith S, et al. Health spending projections through 2018: recession effects add uncertainty to the outlook. *Health Aff (Millwood)*. 2009;28:w346–w357.

13. Orszag PR. CBO Testimony, Peter R. Orszag. Growth in health care costs. Washington, DC: Committee on the Budget, United States Senate; 2008.

14. Chalkidou K, Tunis S, Lopert R, et al. Comparative effectiveness research and evidence-based health policy: experience from four countries. *Milbank Q*. 2009;87:339–367.

15. Orszag PR. Research on the comparative effectiveness of medical treatments from the Congressional Budget Office. Washington, DC: Committee on the Budget, United States Senate; 2007.

16. Wilensky GR. Developing a center for comparative effectiveness information. *Health Aff (Millwood)*. 2006;25:w572–w585.

17. Institute of Medicine. Learning What Works Best: *The Nations Need for Evidence on Comparative Effectiveness in Health Care*. Washington, DC: Institute of Medicine; 2007.

18. Wilensky GR. The policies and politics of creating a comparative clinical effectiveness research center. *Health Aff (Millwood)*. 2009;28:w719–w729.

Index

W

Web-based antidepressant self-monitoring program, 86–89, 91, 94, 97, 100

weight
  assigned, in decision tables, 154–155
  preference, 189

WHI. *See* Women's Health Initiative

WHO. *See* World Health Organization

wholesale price, 172

willingness to pay (WTP), 184, 186, 187, 192

withdrawal, from randomized clinical trials, 100–102

Women's Health Initiative (WHI), 86

World Health Organization (WHO), 26

World Medical Association, 94, 95

World War II, medical experiments during, 94

WTP. *See* willingness to pay

Z

Zantac, 21